TREAT YOUR OWN
KNEE

ROBIN McKENZIE
CNZM, OBE, FCSP (Hon), FNZSP (Hon),
Dip MDT, Dip MT

with Grant Watson
NZSP, ADP (OMT), Dip MT, Dip MDT

and Robert Lindsay
NZSP, ADP (OMT), Dip MT

Spinal Publications New Zealand Limited
Email: info@spinalpublications.co.nz
Telephone: + 64 4 299-7020

ISBN: 978-0-9876504-8-1

Designed by OPTP.
www.optp.com

Photography by Dewey Koshenina, Gamut One Studios.
www.gamut1studios.com

Illustrations by Jono Smith.

Stock Photography from istockphoto.com, shutterstock.com, thinkstock.com

Acknowledgements

The authors would like to thank:

Richard Rosedale and Rob Hughes for contributing their extensive expertise in the McKenzie Method® to the information in this book, and to them and Rowley Watson for assistance with early drafts of the manuscript. We would also like to thank OPTP for their organization of the photo shoot, and Greg Lynch for final proofreading.

We would like to acknowledge the encouragement and guidance of Rachel Mason of Spinal Publications New Zealand Limited, and the creative expertise of our designer, Kirsten Revell and illustrator, Jono Smith, who made the final stages of this book preparation a pleasure.

Finally, we would like to thank the thousands of patients who unknowingly provided most of the solutions for knee pain that are described in this book.

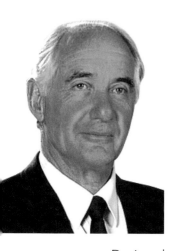

About the Authors

The late Robin McKenzie was born in Auckland, New Zealand, in 1931. He graduated from the New Zealand School of Physiotherapy in 1952 and, after commencing private practice in Wellington, New Zealand in 1953, he specialized in the treatment of spinal disorders.

During the 1960s, Robin McKenzie developed his own examination and treatment methods, and was recognized internationally as an authority on the diagnosis and treatment of low back pain. The McKenzie Method® of mechanical diagnosis and therapy is now taught and practiced worldwide and has evolved to not only relate to spinal disorders but also the treatment of disorders of the extremities (e.g., shoulders, hips and knees). The success of the McKenzie Method has attracted intense interest from researchers worldwide, and it is the most studied diagnostic and treatment system for back pain at the present time (www.mckenziemdt.org). Clinicians surveyed in the United States voted Robin McKenzie the most influential clinician in their daily work.

In 1982, he was made an Honorary Life Member of the American Physical Therapy Association "in recognition of distinguished and meritorious service to the art and science of physical therapy and to the welfare of mankind." In 1983, he was elected to membership of the International Society for the Study of the Lumbar Spine. In 1984, he was made a Fellow of the American Back Society, and in 1985, he was awarded an Honorary Fellowship of the New Zealand Society of Physiotherapists. In 1987, he was made an Honorary Life Member of the New Zealand Manipulative Therapists Association and, in 1990, an Honorary Fellow of the Chartered Society of Physiotherapists in the United Kingdom.

In the 1990 Queen's Birthday Honours, he was made an Officer of the Most Excellent Order of the British Empire (OBE). In the New Year Honours 2000, Her Majesty Queen Elizabeth II appointed Robin McKenzie to be a Companion of the New Zealand Order of Merit (CNZM).

Grant Watson

Grant Watson is a Senior and International Instructor, and Assistant Director of Education, for the McKenzie Institute International. He has represented the Institute extensively in many corners of the world since 1995. He has been actively involved with education within physiotherapy since 1985 and for many years was an Accredited Physiotherapist to the New Zealand Academy of Sport. He is co-author with Robin McKenzie of *Treat Your Own Shoulder* (2009) and co-author of *Treat Your Own Strains, Sprains and Bruises* (1994).

Robert Lindsay

Robert Lindsay is a Physiotherapist in Private Practice in Coromandel Peninsula, New Zealand with post-graduate qualifications in orthopedic and manipulative physiotherapy. He firmly believes in the role of education and self-treatment within the scope of physiotherapy, as people generally are able to successfully treat and prevent or limit recurrence of many of the soft tissue disorders that occur in daily life. He is co-author with Robin McKenzie of *Treat Your Own Shoulder* (2009) and co-author of *Treat Your Own Strains, Sprains and Bruises* (1994).

Books by Robin McKenzie

Mobilization of the Spinal Column
Kaltenborn, F.M. Technical translation by McKenzie, R.
Wellington, N.Z.: New Zealand University Press, Price Milburn, 1970.

Treat Your Own Back™ (9th edition, 2015)
McKenzie, R.
Waikanae, N.Z.: Spinal Publications NZ Ltd, First published 1980.

Treat Your Own Neck™ (5th edition, 2015)
McKenzie, R.
Waikanae, N.Z.: Spinal Publications NZ Ltd, First published 1983.

Treat Your Own Knee™
McKenzie, R. with Watson, G. and Lindsay, R.
Raumati Beach, N.Z.: Spinal Publications NZ Ltd, 2012.

Treat Your Own Shoulder™
McKenzie, R. with Watson, G. and Lindsay, R.
Raumati Beach, N.Z.: Spinal Publications NZ Ltd, 2009.

The Lumbar Spine: Mechanical Diagnosis and Therapy®
(2nd edition, 2003)
McKenzie, R. and May, S.
Waikanae, N.Z.: Spinal Publications NZ Ltd, First published 1981.

The Cervical and Thoracic Spine: Mechanical Diagnosis and Therapy® (2nd edition, 2006)
McKenzie, R and May, S.
Raumati Beach, N.Z.: Spinal Publications NZ Ltd, First published 1990.

The Human Extremities: Mechanical Diagnosis and Therapy®
McKenzie, R and May, S.
Waikanae, N.Z.: Spinal Publications NZ Ltd, 2000.

7 Steps to a Pain-Free Life: How to Rapidly Relieve Back, Neck, and Shoulder Pain (2nd edition, 2014)
McKenzie, R and Kubey, C.
New York: Plume, First published 2001.

Against the Tide: Back pain treatment – the breakthrough: An Autobiography
McKenzie, R with Bybee, R.
Wellington, N.Z.: Dunmore Publishing, 2009.

Contents

Acknowledgements III

About the Authors IV

Books by Robin McKenzie VI

Chapter 1: Introduction 1
Knee problems 1
Osteoarthritis, degeneration or normal wear and tear? 1
Is the pain inevitable? 2
MRI's – do they tell the full story? 2
Myths 3
Is the information in this book suitable for me? 8
Diagnosing your problem 10
Who can perform self-treatment? 12

Chapter 2: Understanding the Knee Region 14
The knee 14
Functions of the knee region 17
Mechanical pain 18
Mechanical knee pain 19
Tissue damage 21

Chapter 3: Common Causes of Knee Pain 22
Consequences of postural neglect 23
1. Inactivity – low fitness levels 24
2. Postural stresses 27
Postural neglect 27
Prolonged sitting postures 28
How to manage prolonged sitting 29
Prolonged standing postures 30
How to manage prolonged standing 30
Lying and sleeping 32
How to manage lying and sleeping 32
3. Being overweight 33
4. Poor biomechanics 34
Anterior knee pain 34

Chapter 4: Understanding the McKenzie Method® 36
The aim of the exercises 36
Effect on pain intensity and location 37
Pain intensity 38
Starting the exercise program 39

Chapter 5: The Exercise Program 40
Overview 40
To start this process of recovery 44
Exercise 1: Active extension in sitting 46
Exercise 2: Knee extension in sitting 48
Exercise 3: Knee extension in standing 50
Exercise 4: Knee flexion in sitting 53
Exercise 5: Knee flexion in standing 55
Exercise 6: Knee flexion in kneeling 57
Review your progress 58
Exercise 7: Knee strengthening in standing,
          two-legged knee bend 61
Exercise 8: Knee strengthening in standing,
          one-legged knee bend 63
When you have no pain or stiffness 66
Recurrence 68

**Chapter 6: Acute Management and Prevention
          of Recurrence** 69
Acute management 69
Prevention of recurrence 71
1. Interrupt prolonged sitting and standing
   postures regularly 73
2. Increase your walking 74
3. Increase your fitness 76
4. Improve your balance 78
5. Weight loss 80
Conclusion 82
References 83
The McKenzie Institute International 84
Licensed Distributors 88

Chapter 1: Introduction

Knee problems

At some time during our lives, many of us will suffer from knee pain. It is one of the most common problems affecting the joints and muscles of the body after back and neck pain, and is the most common site of pain and disability in the upper or lower limbs. The prevalence of people reporting knee pain is around 10% of the 40-50 year-old population, increasing to around 25% of over 70 year-olds. Knee pain quickly affects our ability to do daily tasks like getting up from sitting and squatting or kneeling. Walking or going up and down stairs becomes difficult, and developing a limp can cause pain to develop in other areas as the body tries to compensate.

Osteoarthritis, degeneration or normal wear and tear?

While it is possible to injure our knees by twisting or falling, the most common cause of recurrent knee pain in adults is commonly diagnosed by health professionals as "osteoarthritis." The American Academy of Orthopaedic Surgeons reports that more than 33 million people have osteoarthritis of the knee in the USA. However, this diagnosis is often based almost solely on an X-ray looking for aging changes in the joint, which are evident in up to 70% of the population over 50 years old. But, as in other areas of the body, aging changes on X-ray are not a very accurate guide as to whether pain or disability will be present. The most commonly used term to describe these aging changes is "degeneration" when, in fact, they are usually no more than normal wear and tear. These changes are part of a normal aging process and may not be the cause of pain.

For example, we may complain of pain in one knee joint and find equal aging changes if we X-ray both knees for a comparison. The assumption that this "degeneration" is causing the knee pain becomes very questionable when so many cases start improving in minutes by applying the self-treatment methods described in this book.

Is the pain inevitable?

Similarly, we tend to believe that the pain from osteoarthritis will be slowly progressive and that getting worse is inevitable. However, several studies show that in many people symptoms get no worse or actually improve over time, even as the X-ray changes show deterioration over the same period. This book will give you the information to do everything you can to make that improvement.

MRI's – do they tell the full story?

Magnetic Resonance Imaging (MRI) Scans are another commonly used imaging tool because of their ability to reveal the appearance of damage to the tissues. A commonly injured or damaged structure within the knee is the so-called "cartilage" or "meniscus." Injuries to the meniscus are reported as the second most common injury to the knee. In the USA, 10 to 20% of all orthopedic surgeries consist of surgery to the meniscus on an estimated 850,000 patients each year. However, in many cases, the MRI Scans do not always give us an exact picture of the site or severity of the injury, or give clear guidance for treatment strategies. Many studies show that experts disagree on the interpretation of MRIs, and other studies show that surgeons often find the MRI findings inaccurate when they perform the surgery. While some cases of meniscal injury do require surgery, it has been shown that meniscus surgery increases the risk for future knee surgery by 30%. Studies have shown that up to 76% of older people without knee pain have meniscus damage or tears, and all the Guidelines on Knee Pain around the world recommend avoiding surgery if possible.

Myths

There are many myths associated with aging changes in the knee. The most common of these relate either to the cause:

- "I must have over-used my knee with years of running or hiking for recreation."
- "I have an active occupation and my knees are getting worn out."

Or they relate to management:

- "Now that I have osteoarthritis, I must rest the knee by doing less."
- "Due to my age and pain, I should consider a knee replacement sooner rather than later."

In fact, none of the above are correct. The truth is that most of us are not consistently active enough in our adult lives to maintain the flexibility and strength required for full knee function. A long-term study of runners and non-runners demonstrated no difference in the prevalence of knee osteoarthritis between the two groups, and if you ask around your friends, you will find the same pattern. It is not the more active who consistently report knee pain, but generally the people who have a more sedentary lifestyle. Also, the single most effective management for knee pain of mechanical origin in most people is actually increasing the amount of exercise they give to their knees and gradually increasing overall activity and fitness.

Knee pain can be felt in a variety of ways. There may be some pain or stiffness in both knees although most commonly one knee is more troublesome than the other. There can be days or times in the day when no pain is felt. The symptoms may appear for no apparent reason, and just as mysteriously they disappear or change location. Sometimes the symptoms may only occur with specific movements of the knee, such as getting up from a chair, squatting, kneeling, or walking up and down steps or stairs. At other times, the pain appears when standing or sitting for prolonged periods. These aches and pains may also be felt to some degree at all times throughout the day. It is also common for knee pain to regularly disturb your sleep. People who have pain all of the time are frequently forced to take medication and sometimes have to stop work, or give up certain hobbies, like hiking or golf. The pain simply makes their lives miserable, and they have to reduce their activities in order to keep the discomfort at a manageable level. However, the consequence is that they subsequently start to lose fitness and gain weight, which further impacts their knee problem. Knee problems can thus significantly affect our quality of life.

If you have problems of this nature, you may have already discovered that the symptoms can last for months or even years. You may have found that some treatments decrease or stop your pain temporarily, but the pain returns later when you try to return to your normal activities. You may be reading this book because you have persistent pains that have not disappeared, despite the fact that you may have received many types of treatments.

Common treatments for knee pain are medication, injections, surgery, acupuncture, or electrical modalities such as ultrasound, TENS, or interferential therapy. However, while some of these treatments may appear to give short-term benefit, none have strong evidence that they provide effective long-term relief from pain and loss of function. Similarly, following an extensive review of many studies, the American Academy of Orthopaedic Surgeons does not support the widely advertised nutritional supplements, such as glucosamine or chondroitin sulphate. Although these do no harm, they do not get to the real cause of pain and are no better than placebo treatment in some studies.

You may also have been given exercises to perform, and perhaps you have found these to be of some benefit. However, many people do not realize that stretching and strengthening your muscles alone does not automatically give you relief from knee pain. "Doing your exercises" is only part of the solution. What we seldom consider are the other aggravating factors that contribute to your knee pain. The most important thing for most people is to be more active with walking or other recreational interests, and where indicated, lose some body weight.

Also, it is important to understand how prolonged static positions or postures you adopt during various occupations or activities, such as prolonged standing as a shop assistant or factory worker (Photo 1), or prolonged kneeling or squatting as a tradesman or cleaner (Photo 2) can significantly contribute to your knee problem. Prolonged sitting with your knees bent, as in a sedentary occupation, such as an office worker (Photo 3), or relaxing at home (Photo 4), can also be harmful if these positions are not regularly interrupted.

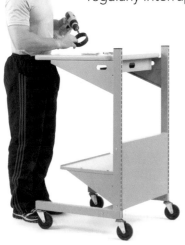

Photo 1 Prolonged standing

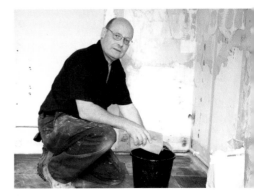

Photo 2 Kneeling

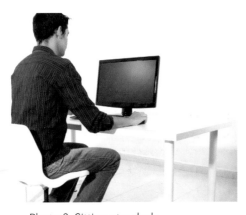

Photo 3 Sitting at a desk

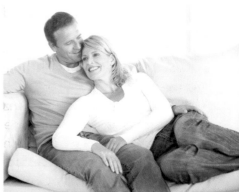

Photo 4 Relaxing

Whatever the situation, you have most likely realized that many of the treatments dispensed by doctors and physical therapists are prescribed for your present symptoms and are not directed at preventing future problems. Time and again you may have to seek assistance to get relief from your knee pain. How satisfying would it be to be able to apply treatment to yourself whenever pain arose? Better still, to apply a system of treatment to yourself that would prevent or reduce the onset of pain?

It has been shown repeatedly that patients require a rational explanation for their problems. They need education about the postures, activities and exercises that allow them to remain free of disabling symptoms. They need advice on how to avoid or manage the detrimental forces encountered in daily living and how to apply beneficial strategies. All of these things are found in this book.

Since the 1970s, methods have been discovered that enable us to understand how to manage our own spinal and extremity problems. The self-treatment methods that we describe to you here evolved after Robin McKenzie's experiences with more than 20,000 patients during 40 years of practice. The methods have been used for back and neck pain by doctors and physical therapists in many parts of the world for decades. Millions of people like you have found relief by reading the first two books in this series, *Treat Your Own Back*, and *Treat Your Own Neck*. More recently, this same McKenzie approach has been used for mechanical pain in other regions of the body, such as the shoulder and knee, and the majority of patients are achieving the same very satisfactory results. This led to the publication of *Treat Your Own Shoulder* in 2009.

One of the main points of this book is that the management of your knee is best accomplished by you. If, for some reason, you have developed knee problems, then you must learn how to deal with the present symptoms and how to prevent or limit future problems. Self-treatment will be more effective in the long-term management of your knee pain than any other form of treatment because you can self-treat multiple times a day. It is the least expensive treatment and safer than receiving treatment from other people. Self-management gives you the tools to get better and stay better.

Is the information in this book suitable for me?

The majority of people will benefit from the advice given in this book, which is provided for those people with straightforward recurring mechanical problems. Nearly everyone can begin the exercise program, provided the recommended precautions are taken as described later in this chapter.

However, in any of the following situations, you should not begin the exercise program without first consulting your doctor or physical therapist:

- If your knee has suddenly become very swollen or hot for no apparent reason, or you think it may have become infected.

- If you are generally feeling unwell in conjunction with your knee pain.

- If you have associated back pain, with pain or numbness radiating to the front of the thigh and/or the knee region.

- If you have severe pain in the leg below the knee and experience sensations of weakness, numbness or pins and needles in the foot.

- If you have developed severe pain in the back of the leg below the knee with associated chest pain or breathlessness.

- If you have suddenly developed severe knee pain following a recent accident and find you are unable to take any weight through your leg or it keeps collapsing or "locking" for no reason.

- If you have a previous history of cancer or a tumor.

- If you have had knee surgery in the past three months.

If you have developed knee pain for the first time, you must follow the instructions and guidelines over the next several pages even more carefully. If you have any doubt about your suitability for the information in this book, we recommend you consult your doctor or physical therapist for advice and treatment, and instructions on the prevention of further knee problems.

Choose your clinician carefully. You should be provided with the information and education you require to manage your own problem. Every patient deserves to have the opportunity to learn how to manage their own knee problem, and every clinician should be obligated to provide that information. This is the essence of the McKenzie Method®.

The only healthcare professionals fully qualified to provide the McKenzie Method are members of the McKenzie Institute International who hold the credentialing certificate or the Diploma in Mechanical Diagnosis & Therapy®. A clinician in your area can be located via the McKenzie Institute International website www.mckenziemdt.org.

We recommend you carefully follow the guidelines and instructions in the rest of this chapter to assess your suitability for this program, or to establish whether you should consult a health professional first. The information provided will enable you to determine with reasonable certainty whether your knee is the source of your pain and if you will benefit from the methods outlined in this book.

Once you have started the exercises, carefully watch your pain pattern. If your pains are getting progressively worse and remain worse the following day, or if they are slowly increasing in severity and becoming intolerable, you should seek advice from your doctor or a McKenzie Institute International credentialed or diplomaed clinician to learn alternative exercises or to consider other treatment strategies.

Diagnosing your problem

Chapter 2 will discuss the anatomy and workings of the knee region to help you to understand your knee problem. However, let us consider the behavior of your pain at this point.

Pain location

As a general rule, knee pain or aching when of mechanical origin will be felt within the knee and may be associated with stiffness or weakness. It may be felt more in one particular spot, or it may change location from side to side, or in front or at the back of the knee.

This general knee pain may on occasion radiate down toward the upper shin area (Figure 1), but it is very uncommon for affected knee structures to cause pain to be felt above the knee, or to radiate upward into the hip or back regions (Figure 2).

However, it is possible for back or hip pain to radiate downward toward the knee, and even into the foot (Figure 3). Similarly, a knee problem will not give you a sensation of pins and needles, or numbness, in the leg or foot. These symptoms are much more likely to be referred from the low back.

Some people report that their knee pain is very specific to the front part of the knee around the region of the knee cap or patella. Often this condition is referred to as **anterior knee pain**, and is covered in more detail in Chapter 3. Many readers classified with this condition will be able to effectively self-treat and manage their pain by following the information in this book.

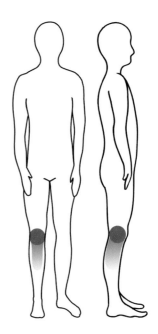

Figure 1

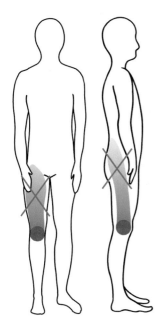

Figure 2

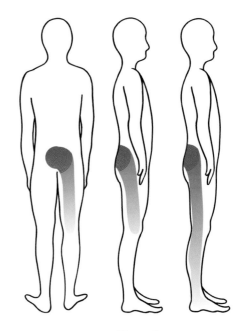

Figure 3

Who can perform self-treatment?

Having determined that your knee region is the source of your pain, we recommend you spend a further couple of minutes completing the following checklist. Answering all the questions will determine whether you can treat your knee successfully without further assistance:

	Yes	No
• Are there periods in the day when you have no pain or aching? Even ten minutes?	☐	☐
• Do you have pain when you walk up or down stairs or hills?	☐	☐
• Have you had several episodes of knee pain over the past months or years?	☐	☐
• Between episodes, is your knee pain-free?	☐	☐
• When the knee is painful, does it feel like you are unable to fully bend or straighten it compared to your pain-free knee?	☐	☐
• Between episodes, are you able to fully bend and straighten your knee without pain?	☐	☐
• Is the pain localized to the area of the knee joint?	☐	☐
• Between your episodes of knee pain, are you generally able to walk without limping?	☐	☐
• Are you generally worse with prolonged sitting, squatting or kneeling?	☐	☐
• Is your knee generally more comfortable when you are moving about rather than kneeling, sitting, squatting or standing in one position?	☐	☐
• Are some days better or worse than others?	☐	☐

If you answered:

- **'Yes' to all of the previous questions,** you are an ideal candidate for the self-treatment outlined in this book.

- **'Yes' to five or more questions,** your chances to benefit from self-treatment are good and you should begin the program.

- **'Yes' to only four or fewer questions,** then some form of specialized treatment may be required and you should consult a clinician credentialed or diplomaed by the McKenzie Institute International. A clinician in your area can be located via the McKenzie Institute International website: www.mckenziemdt.org.

This book describes a complete system of management, which must be followed in its entirety to ensure success. Do not turn straight to the exercise description pages; your understanding of chapters 1-4 is essential.

Chapter 2: Understanding the Knee Region

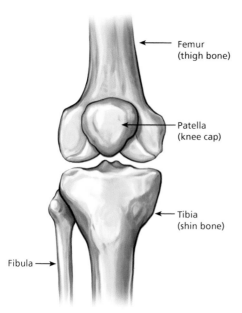

Femur
(thigh bone)

Patella
(knee cap)

Tibia
(shin bone)

Fibula

Figure 4
Right knee

The knee

The knee is a hinge joint between the thigh bone, the femur, and the shin bone, known as the tibia. A narrower shin bone called the fibula lies parallel on the outer side of the tibia. In front of the knee joint is the knee cap or patella. This oval-shaped bone sits within the quadriceps tendon and improves the mechanics of the quadriceps muscle over the front of the knee (Figure 4).

The joint surfaces of the femur, tibia and patella, which form the knee joint, are covered with a substance called articular cartilage, which gives a smooth protective coating to the joint, similar to the surface of a ball bearing. Within the knee joint, between the femur and the tibia are two cartilage cushions, known as menisci, which help distribute the load of the femur evenly on the tibia.

The knee joint itself is surrounded by a sack-like structure called a capsule, which assists in supporting the knee joint. It also contains the lubricating fluid that circulates through the knee joint to assist with its nutrition.

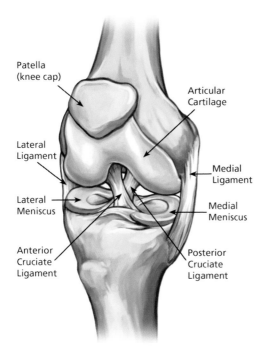

Patella
(knee cap)

Articular
Cartilage

Lateral
Ligament

Medial
Ligament

Lateral
Meniscus

Medial
Meniscus

Anterior
Cruciate
Ligament

Posterior
Cruciate
Ligament

Figure 5
Right knee

For further support, the knee joint relies on four strap-like bands called ligaments to hold the joint together and guide movement. The ligament located on the inner side of the knee is known as the medial ligament, and the ligament on the outer side of the knee the lateral ligament. These two ligaments provide side-to-side support and stability. Within the knee itself are the other two ligaments known as the anterior, and the posterior, cruciate ligaments. The role of these two ligaments is to limit forward and backward movement of the tibia on the femur (Figure 5). All these knee ligaments are very strong, and although they may be strained or even occasionally ruptured in a serious knee injury, this usually occurs in a high-impact sports situation, such as football or skiing.

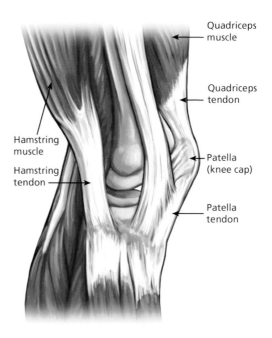

Quadriceps
muscle

Quadriceps
tendon

Hamstring
muscle

Hamstring
tendon

Patella
(knee cap)

Patella
tendon

Figure 6
Right knee

Two main muscle groups create movement at the knee,
with cord-like structures called tendons crossing the joint.
The hamstring muscle group is located at the back of
the thigh and works when you lift your heel toward your
buttocks. The quadriceps muscle group is located on
the front of the thigh and contracts when you straighten
your leg when performing an activity such as climbing a
hill or stairs, or acts as a brake, slowly releasing during
activities such as sitting down or going down a hill or
stairs (Figure 6). The quadriceps tendon, patella, and
patella tendon absorb a great deal of force during
weight bearing movement at the knee and sometimes
can become a source of knee pain. This condition is
known as anterior knee pain and is discussed further
in chapter 3.

Functions of the knee region

The design of the knee supports our body weight and allows strength and power for the performance of a range of physical tasks, such as rising from sitting (Photo 5), lifting and carrying heavy loads (Photo 6), climbing or descending steps (Photo 7) and running (Photo 8). However, the knee is also vulnerable to twisting or sideways forces or strains, which can damage the joint surfaces, a meniscus, or the ligaments.

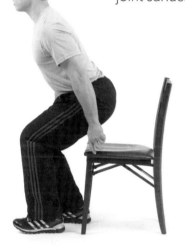

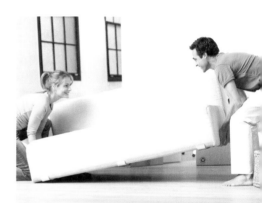

Photo 5 Rising from sitting

Photo 6 Lifting heavy loads

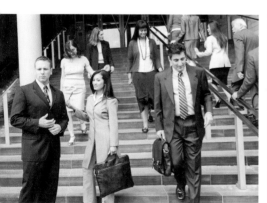

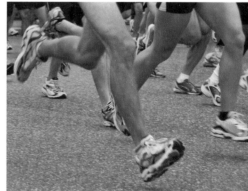

Photo 7 Climbing or descending stairs

Photo 8 Running

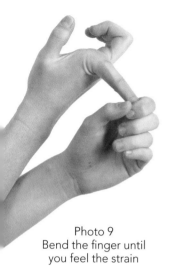

Mechanical pain

Pain of mechanical origin occurs when a pain-sensitive structure is overstretched, overloaded or compressed — either by a single significant event, such as a blow or twist; or repeated actions, such as running downhill; or over a sustained duration, such as prolonged standing or squatting. This is true for mechanical pain in any region of the body, including the knee. To help you understand how easily some mechanical pains can be produced, you may like to try a simple experiment. First, bend one finger backward until you feel a strain, as shown in Photo 9.

Photo 9
Bend the finger until
you feel the strain

If you keep your finger in this position, you initially feel only minor discomfort, but as time passes, pain eventually develops. In some cases, pain caused by prolonged stretching or compressive forces may take as much as an hour to be felt.

Try the experiment once more, but now keep bending the finger past the point of strain until you feel the immediate sensation of pain. You have overstretched, and your pain warning system is telling you that to continue movement in that particular direction will cause damage.

The pain warning tells you to stop overstretching to avoid damage and, when you do so, the pain ceases immediately. No damage has occurred and the pain has gone. No lasting problems arise from this short-lived strain providing you take note of the pain warning system.

If you fail to heed the warning and keep the finger in the overstretched position, the ligaments and surrounding soft tissues that hold the joint together will eventually overstretch and tear. This tearing will result in an ache that continues even when you stop overstretching. The discomfort or pain reduces in intensity but continues even when the finger is at rest. The pain increases with movement performed in the direction that overstretches the affected tissues and will not cease until some healing has occurred. Healing may take several days, but would be prolonged if every day you were to continue to apply the same strains to the finger. The same things happen when you overstretch the structures in and around your knee.

Mechanical knee pain

In the knee region, the knee ligaments, menisci, capsule, and surrounding tendons are responsible for supporting the knee joint and allowing movement to occur. Mechanical knee pain often arises due to overstretching, overloading or distorting these tissues. This may occur without further damage, as in the bent finger example on the previous page. Overstretching may be caused by a force placing a sudden severe strain on the knee, for example, a sudden twist (Photo 10) or a fall (Photo 11) onto the knee. This type of stress cannot easily be avoided as it occurs unexpectedly.

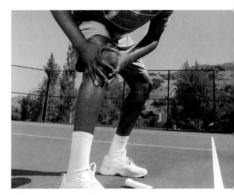

Photo 10 Sudden twist

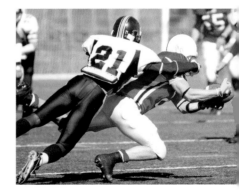

Photo 11 A fall

However, more often overstretching or overloading is caused by postural stresses that place less severe strains on the knee over a longer time period. Examples include performing work or activities where you are standing in the same position for a prolonged period of time; or performing an activity with either repeated or sustained bent leg positions, such as kneeling or squatting — for example, changing a car tire (Photo 12) — or sitting with your knees bent more than 120 degrees (Photo 13). In some cases, pain caused by prolonged standing or sitting may take as long as an hour to appear.

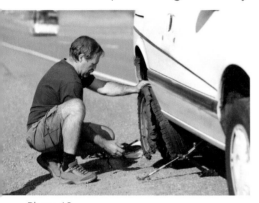

Photo 12
Sustained bent leg

By understanding the potential for injury in repeatedly performing these actions or sustaining the bent leg posture for prolonged periods of time, we can learn to minimize these adverse loads on our knees. Herein lies one of our main responsibilities in the self-treatment and prevention of knee pain.

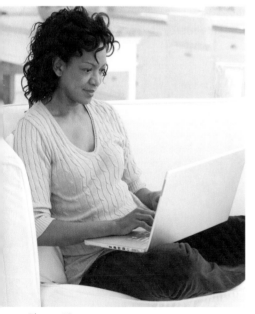

Photo 13
Knees bent more than 120 degrees

Tissue damage

Complications arise when overstretching or overloading of soft tissues around the knee leads to actual tissue damage. It is often thought that knee pain is caused by strained muscles. This is not the case. Muscles, which are the source of power and movement, can be overstretched but usually heal rapidly and seldom cause pain lasting more than a week or two.

The real problem is the knee joint itself and its associated soft tissue structures, which may be injured from overstretching or overloading. Pain from these injured structures will interfere with the normal muscle function, particularly the quadriceps muscle group, resulting in the muscles weakening. This further reduces the strength and function of the knee and makes the structures of the knee more vulnerable to further damage.

These damaged structures undergo a healing process that may result in an incomplete repair, and become less elastic and weakened. Once soft tissues are damaged, pain is felt until healing is complete and function is fully restored. In most cases, the solution for these pain-sensitive structures is to remodel the affected tissues by gradually applying progressive forces and avoiding or modifying the adverse loading on these affected structures. Unless appropriate exercises are performed to gradually stretch and strengthen these structures and restore their normal flexibility and function, they will become a continuous source of knee pain. In frustration, some people turn to injections or even surgery that may not be necessary.

Chapter 3: Common causes of knee pain

There are several structures within the knee region that can give rise to knee pain. These are the capsule and ligaments, which hold the joint together; and the menisci, joint surfaces and underlying bone, which are the load bearing components of the knee joint itself as discussed in Chapter 2.

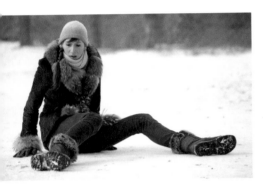

Photo 14 Slipping on a wet surface

The knee is also vulnerable to twisting or sideways forces or strains, which can damage the joint surfaces, a meniscus, or the ligaments. These structures may be injured and, in the case of ligaments and menisci, even torn when we wrench our knee performing a forceful twisting action, particularly when the foot is fixed on the ground. Common events could be slipping on a wet surface (Photo 14), during sport (Photo 15), or receiving a direct blow, such as falling onto your knees (Photo 16).

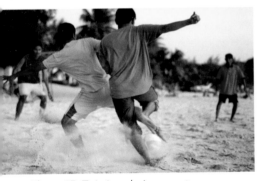

Photo 15 Twisting during sport

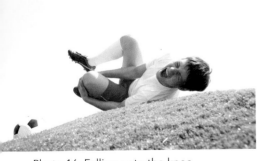

Photo 16 Falling onto the knee

IF YOU ARE READING THIS BOOK FOR THE FIRST
TIME AND HAVE JUST INJURED YOUR KNEE IN THIS
WAY (WITHIN ONE TO TWO DAYS), SEE THE SECTION
ON ACUTE MANAGEMENT ON PAGE 69 IN CHAPTER 6
FOR INFORMATION ON HOW TO MANAGE A RECENT
SOFT TISSUE INJURY TO THE KNEE.

Consequences of postural neglect

However, a specific injury or incident, as described on
the previous page, is not the only cause of injuries to
the knee. If we sustain static positions for long periods
and only apply load sporadically through a small range
of motion, as is common in our adult lives, the knee joint
gradually becomes less able to tolerate the peaks of load
when we increase the loading on the knee too quickly.
This can occur with a rapid increase in repetitive activities,
such as walking or running, or performing actions that
produce a sudden increased load on the knee, such as
a jump or deep squat. The joint surfaces are vulnerable
to damage when the shock-absorbing capabilities of
the structures in and around the knee are overloaded.

It is this combination of normal aging changes, gradual
deterioration of a healthy joint through lack of use, and
associated injuries along the way that contribute to the
development of knee pain as the smooth cartilage
erodes and the menisci and other soft tissues become
pain sensitive.

If we lose the full range of painless motion and functional
strength through the development of a painful knee, it
quickly impacts our daily life and can affect everyday tasks
such as walking, using stairs, crouching, prolonged sitting
and work or recreational activities.

Like the other joints in the body, our knees require regular controlled movement and activity to nourish and maintain the structures in and around the knee to enable a high level of pain-free function.

Therefore, the most common causes of developing and prolonging knee pain are much less obvious and relate to four main factors:

1. Inactivity — low fitness levels
2. Postural stresses — prolonged standing or sitting
3. Being overweight
4. Poor biomechanics

1. Inactivity — low fitness levels

In our so-called "modern" lifestyles, the great majority of us simply don't do enough general exercise for our knees. Our legs are designed for walking, running, climbing and jumping — but we spend little time doing these. Mostly, we fold our legs underneath us seated at a table or desk. Many of us have sedentary occupations where we sit most of the day, often at computers or driving (Photo 17). Then at home most of us sit for prolonged periods in the evenings watching TV, eating a meal, or back at the computer (Photo 18). A recent study in Britain indicated that on average adults spend 14 hours a day sitting.

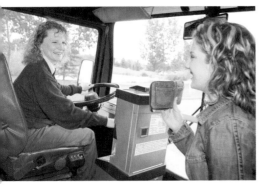

Photo 17 Sedentary occupation

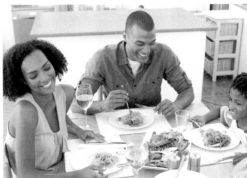

Photo 18 Sedentary lifestyle

It is no coincidence that many people develop recurrent and persistent knee pain in their thirties to forties. This is the onset of "middle age" when we gradually begin to exercise less, and it is the age when our body's metabolism changes and we have a tendency to put on weight. Additionally, it is the age when the tissues of the body begin to become less flexible and lose the capacity to absorb adverse load. Between the ages of 50-70, we lose about 30% of our strength from disuse. The average 20-year-old uses 20% of their capacity to rise from a chair; the average 70-year-old uses 90%. Often knee pain causes avoidance of activities that strengthen the legs, such as stair climbing.

Think back to when you were a child, and remember how active you once were, or simply observe a group of children. It is very difficult for them to sit for any length of time as their natural inclination is to be on the move. Then, when we do encourage them to have a break, what do they do? They invariably get up and run around, or hop, jump or skip. All the time they are using the joints and muscles of their legs, and developing the endurance and strength to perform increasing amounts of sustained physical activity.

Contrast that to ourselves as adults. It is very unusual for us to be on the move for any length of time, and our natural inclination is to get back to sitting as soon as possible. **What do you do in your lunch break at work after sitting all morning? Most likely you walk a few steps and then sit again for the majority of your break.** Similarly, our city and urban communities, with shopping malls and public buildings, provide us with all sorts of facilities that minimize the amount of walking we have to do.

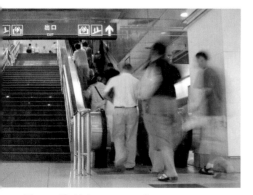

Photo 19 Using an escalator instead of the stairs

We drive our cars or take public transport as close as possible to our destination, we use escalators or elevators, and we sit on the available stools, benches or chairs provided at every opportunity (Photo 19).

Low levels of fitness cause us to avoid activities because we get out of breath. But as fitness declines further, our body weight, and the corresponding load on the knees, tends to increase.

The knee joint and its surrounding muscles respond to appropriate exercise and load. Regularly loading the knee with physical activity assists with the nutrition within the knee and keeps the surrounding muscles flexible and strong, which in turn maintains the knee's sense of balance and coordination. Conversely the opposite is true, if we don't keep active and we don't put our knees through a full range of movement, they gradually lose range of motion. This contributes to losing muscle strength and decreasing our tolerance to perform sustained levels of physical activity. This loss of movement and strength contributes to mechanical pain as well as making our knee more susceptible to the sudden twisting or impact stresses described at the start of this chapter.

However, there is very good evidence in the medical literature for increasing our general activity to reverse this decline in the strength and function of our knees. Also, many studies have shown that this "training" effect on the body's tissues occurs even well into older age if the loading is graduated and regular. It is never too late to get more active, providing you start gently. Chapter 6 describes simple ideas and effective strategies to assist you with a graduated increase in your activities to improve and maintain your knee function.

2. Postural stresses

In addition to the problems caused by inactivity, there are some specific knee positions that contribute to excess stress on the joint structures. These stresses arise from prolonged or repeated activities that can adversely load the knee joint structures.

The common postures and prolonged positions we adopt that affect the structures of the knee are primarily a combination of these three factors:

- Performing repetitive or prolonged tasks with our knees bent while taking some load on the knee. For example, prolonged crouching or kneeling without taking regular breaks from this position. Also, in some cases, prolonged sitting in a low chair with bent knees and our feet on the floor results in an adverse load through the anterior structures of the knee that can produce significant knee pain.

- Standing still for an extended period of time places a prolonged static load through the joint surfaces without the opportunity for them to have any time to recover in an unloaded position.

- Lying and sleeping with a knee positioned incorrectly can place either direct pressure or an inappropriate postural stress on the affected structures of the knee.

Postural Neglect

When these postures are maintained long enough, they cause overstretching or overloading of the structures in and around the knee. Thus pain will arise only in certain positions. Knee problems developed in this way are the consequence of postural neglect. Sustained knee posture is not the only cause of knee pain.

However, once knee problems have developed, sustained postures will frequently make them worse and perpetuate them. Some people who habitually adopt poor knee postures and remain unaware of the underlying cause experience knee pain throughout their adult lifetime simply because they were not in possession of the necessary information to correct the postural faults.

Pains of postural origin are often first felt as a minor irritation and are easily ignored, as they are eliminated merely by correcting the postures. However, as time passes, these uncorrected habitual knee or leg postures cause changes to the structures of the knee. Excessive wear occurs, with loss of elasticity resulting in changes to the structures in and around the knee. When this occurs, pain becomes more frequent and persistent. The effects of poor posture and general inactivity in the long-term, therefore, can be just as severe and harmful as the effects of injury.

Should pain develop, there are certain movements or posture modifications you can perform in order to stop that pain. You should not have to seek assistance whenever postural pain arises.

Prolonged sitting postures

You may have been sitting with bent knees for many years without knee pain. However, consistently sitting with your knee bent in one position for a period of time, for example, at a cramped work station, will gradually cause an over-stretching and over-loading of the structures in and around the knee. You will often find your knee is initially stiff and uncomfortable as you stand up from the prolonged sitting position. If you continue to persist with the static bent knee posture, your knee will become painful in the sitting position as well as when you rise from sitting. If you already have knee pain you will have probably noticed how bent knee sitting aggravates your pain.

How to manage prolonged sitting

If your knee pain is either produced or aggravated by prolonged sitting, it is important to correct the posture that is causing the pain. Maintaining a bent knee posture will only perpetuate the overloading discussed previously. As a general rule, avoid sitting with your knee bent more than ninety degrees (Photo 20), and if you cannot place your feet flat on the floor, use a foot stool as recommended in good work space design. If you are unable to avoid prolonged sitting with your knees bent in one position for prolonged periods, regularly straighten and bend your affected knee, particularly as soon as you feel any symptoms. Every thirty minutes, perform this simple exercise: Sit upright in your chair and straighten your leg for five seconds; then perform the same exercise with your other leg (Photo 21). Perform the exercise five times for each leg. If you do not have the space to move your leg, it will be necessary to take a regular break from your activity to stand up and go for a short walk. At every refreshment break ensure you go for a walk of at least a few minutes if possible to allow your knee to recover from being bent in one position.

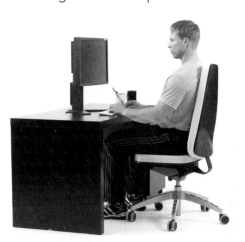

Photo 20 Avoid sitting with knee bent over 90 degrees

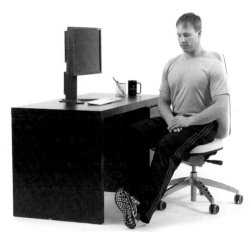

Photo 21 Regularly straighten your leg

Prolonged standing postures

When you stand in one position for long enough, your affected knee will start to feel uncomfortable from the static loading you have placed through the joint. You may take a few steps to ease the discomfort but the pain will return once you return to a static standing position again. If you are standing on a concrete floor or wearing footwear that does not have a cushioning sole, the onset of knee pain is likely to occur sooner.

As time passes, this sustained standing in one position can cause changes to the weight-bearing structures within the knee. The joint surfaces will lose their shock-absorbing capacity and become painful when you are standing for any duration.

How to manage prolonged standing

If you have developed knee pain from standing still for prolonged periods, it is necessary for you to remove this adverse postural stress on your knee by sitting down and performing the following exercise every thirty minutes. Start by sitting upright in a firm chair or stool (Photo 22) with your feet flat on the floor. If you sit forward on the edge of the chair and lean backward you will find it easier to perform this exercise. Slowly bend your knee up toward you (Photo 23), and with both hands pull up on your leg just above your ankle. Slowly pull your heel toward your buttock until you feel a firm tension at your knee (Photo 24). Hold for a few seconds; then return your knee to the starting position. Repeat five times. Now repeat the exercise five times for your other knee to try and prevent the onset of knee pain.

At each refreshment break, go for a short walk; if that is not possible, "march on the spot." If your knee pain continues, you will find it necessary to sit on a chair or stool to unload your knee.

Prolonged standing on a concrete floor places more stress on the knee than standing on a wooden floor. Supportive footwear with a cushion sole will also assist in reducing the adverse load being placed on your knees. Cushioning mats for standing will also be helpful.

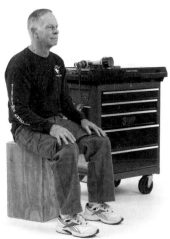

Photo 22 Sit upright

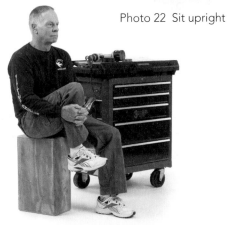

Photo 23 Bend sore knee

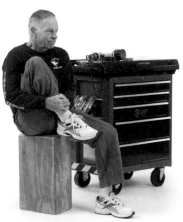

Photo 24 Pull heel toward hip

CHAPTER 3 **Common causes of knee pain**   31

Lying and sleeping

If you wake up in the morning with a painful knee that was not causing problems the night before, or your knee pain wakes you consistently during the night, it is likely there is something wrong with the position of your knee when you sleep. If you are lying in a position that is placing an adverse stress on your knee, either by lying on your side with your knees pressed together or lying with your knee in the fully extended or bent position, a gradual overloading or overstretching of the painful structures occurs. Thus poor sleeping postures can further aggravate an already painful knee.

How to manage lying and sleeping

There are two things to consider with knee pain from lying or sleeping. If you lie on your side with your knees pressed together (Photo 25), this will place a compressive load and often can only be tolerated for a short period before you have to change position. Many people find lying on their side with a pillow between their knees (Photo 26) takes some of the load off the affected knee. It is also necessary to avoid lying with your affected knee either bent up past ninety degrees or fully straightened out, as these positions will place adverse postural stresses on your knee. If this does not provide relief, it is recommended you sleep on your back with a pillow under your knee (Photo 27) to provide support, as this also avoids placing your knee in the fully extended position.

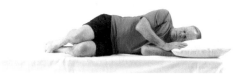

Photo 25 Lying on side with knees pressed together

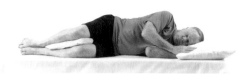

Photo 26 Lying on side with pillow between knees

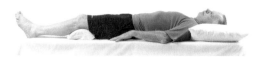

Photo 27 Sleeping on back with pillow under knee

3. Being overweight

As mentioned briefly in Chapter 1, the American Academy of Orthopaedic Surgeons (AAOS) clearly links being overweight to the onset of knee pain in adults, and this is not just an American phenomenon. Many of us gradually put on excess weight through our middle years — again mostly as a result of our modern lifestyles where food is readily available and affordable. But we also find it harder at this stage of our lives to find the time and the desire to exercise sufficiently.

A commonly used formula to approximately measure the percentage of body fat is the Body Mass Index or BMI. It is defined as the individual's body weight divided by the square of his or her height — kg/m^2, or $(lbs./inches^2) \times 703$. An average BMI is approximately 20–30. Numerous studies have confirmed that having a body mass index over 25 points is associated with increased risk of knee pain and associated loss of function. There is also an increased likelihood of developing other health problems, such as diabetes, high blood pressure, heart attacks and a shortened lifespan. It is easy to measure your BMI to determine whether you are overweight. If you go online and search "bmi calculator" you will find a number of websites that will do the calculation for you once you enter your height, weight and age.

The AAOS Knee Guidelines also identify 25 as an appropriate baseline and recommend 5% weight loss for anybody with a BMI greater than 25 if osteoarthritis changes are evident on X-ray (that is most of us in our forties and fifties and above). It has shown that a modest loss in weight results in a significant decrease in knee pain, and in most cases 5% would appear to be a reasonable target. For many people this can be achieved over a few weeks or months by eating less or differently with an appropriate weight loss regime and exercising more. Some simple advice and strategies for weight loss and increasing general exercise are covered further in Chapter 6.

However, we recommend you seek advice from your doctor or physician, or attend a recognized weight loss program, should you have underlying health issues or seek to lose a significant amount of weight.

4. Poor biomechanics

Biomechanics is the name given to the science concerned with the internal and external forces acting on the human body and the effects produced by these forces. In simple terms, poor biomechanics relate to uneven load bearing of the knee caused by the position of the feet and the angle of the knee joints in relation to the feet and the pelvic region.

When we consider knee pain, there is some evidence that poor biomechanics can cause adverse loads on the knee in a small number of people, contributing to and prolonging knee pain. In some cases, suitable footwear with an orthotic inner sole can alter the mechanics of the knee and reduce the pain. This is particularly true for some people with anterior knee pain.

Anterior knee pain

One relatively common and frustrating source of knee pain is pain that is felt only at the front of the knee — usually behind or at the lower aspect of the knee cap. One knee may be affected in isolation, but commonly both knees will be affected to some extent.

This painful condition is generally called anterior knee pain because of the uncertainty about a specific cause, and therefore there is also uncertainty about the best treatment options. Variations of the condition are also referred to as Chondromalacia Patellae, or Patello-Femoral Syndrome (PFS).

Generally it is recognized that excessive repetitive forces on the knee joint region can affect the posture of the patella statically or dynamically and cause adverse load through the patello-femoral joint. Patella Tendonosis, or "jumper's knee," is a more specific cause related to the patella tendon and its attachment to the lower part of the patella.

The factors causing anterior knee pain are not fully understood. Losing the flexibility, strength and coordination in the muscles around the knee can be contributing factors, and less commonly, the faulty mechanics listed on the previous page may also be relevant. The condition frequently affects people in their late teens or early twenties and women more than men, and the problem may continue for many years. Often anterior knee pain comes on for no apparent reason, but sometimes it is associated with a sudden increase in a new activity, such as a sport that involves sudden changes in direction or jumping, or hiking in hill country. A fall onto the front of the knee or prolonged kneeling may also contribute.

People with anterior knee pain frequently find that their knee has a full range of motion with no obstruction to movement compared to the other leg. The pain is usually produced or made worse with prolonged sitting with bent knees, squatting, or performing an aggravating activity, such as walking down stairs or hills, or playing their chosen sport.

Conventional treatments often have a lack of long-term success, and therefore the emphasis needs to be placed on the person to apply effective ongoing self-treatment. The information regarding appropriate knee positions and activity modifications in this chapter will be an important part in minimizing and managing your anterior knee pain. Chapter 5 (page 40) will explain how to determine if your anterior knee pain will benefit from the treatment described in this book and give guidance as to when to seek further advice from a healthcare professional.

Chapter 4: Understanding the McKenzie Method®

The aim of the exercises

The aim of the exercises is to abolish pain and, where appropriate, to restore normal function — that is, to regain full mobility and strength in the knee or as much movement as possible under the given circumstances.

When you are exercising for **pain relief**, you should move **just into the pain**, release the pressure and return to the starting position. As you release the stretch, the pain must diminish back to the starting level or less. If it does not, you are overdoing it and must use less force on your next attempt. When you are exercising for **stiffness**, the exercises can be made more effective by firmly and steadily applying overpressure (as described in Chapter 5) in order to obtain the maximum amount of movement. In this case, a feeling of discomfort may persist afterward, but not for more than 20 minutes or you are overdoing it and need to apply less pressure next time.

Maintenance of correct knee postures and positions should always occur following the exercises. Once you no longer have knee pain, ongoing good postural habits are essential to prevent the recurrence of knee pain.

Effect on pain intensity and location

There are three main effects to look for while performing the exercises:

1. They may cause the symptoms to disappear.

2. They may cause an increase or decrease in the intensity of the pain that you experience.

3. They may cause the pain to move from where you usually feel it to some other location.

In certain cases, the symptoms first change location, then they reduce in intensity and finally they cease altogether.

The effects of exercise on intensity or location of pain can sometimes be very rapid. It is possible to reduce the intensity or change the location of pain after completing as few as 10 movements, and in some conditions, the pain can completely disappear.

In order to determine whether the exercise program is beneficial for you, it is very important that you observe closely any changes in the location of the pain. You may notice that pain, originally felt on the back, front or one side of your knee, moves to a different location in your knee as a result of the exercises.

Pain intensity

If your knee pain is of such intensity that you can only move your leg with difficulty and cannot find a position to lie comfortably in bed, your approach to the exercises should be cautious and unhurried.

On attempting any of the exercises, you may experience an initial increase in pain. This is common and can be expected. As you continue to practice, the pain should quickly diminish, at least to its former level. Usually this occurs during the first exercise session. This will often be followed by the pain becoming more localized to one area of the knee joint. Once the pain becomes localized, the intensity of the pain will generally steadily decrease over a period of a few days, and by continuing the exercises the pain will often disappear entirely.

If, following an initial pain increase, the pain continues to increase in intensity or spreads to places farther away from the knee, such as farther down the leg into your calf muscle or up to the thigh, you should stop exercising and seek professional advice. In other words, do not continue with any of the exercises if your symptoms are much worse immediately after exercising and **remain worse the next day**; or if, during exercising, symptoms are produced or increased in the leg below the knee.

As discussed earlier, once you have started this exercise program, you should expect new exercise pains to develop. These are different from your original pain and are usually felt in areas of the knee that were previously not affected. New pains are the result of performing work your body is not used to and, provided you continue with the exercises, they will wear off in three to four days.

If your symptoms have been present rather continuously for many weeks or months, you should not expect to be pain-free in two to three days. The response will be slower, but if you are doing the correct exercises, it will only be a matter of time before the pain subsides.

As long as your pain is slowly improving, continue with the exercise program that has led to this improvement. Do not change anything in your newly established routine, including no change to pain medication at first. It may be tempting to add other exercises, but this may disrupt your progress. Wait until improvement stops or your pain is 75% better before progressing your exercise program or considering a cautious start with any other activity or exercise.

Starting the exercise program

When you start this exercise program you should stop any other exercise that you may have been shown elsewhere or you happen to do regularly for fitness or sport. If you want to continue with exercises other than the ones described in this book for knee problems, you should wait until your pains have subsided completely.

Chapter 5: The Exercise Program

Overview

In the opening chapters, we have outlined the conditions that can cause pain, reduce mobility and limit function in your knee. As discussed in Chapter 1, it is sometimes difficult to determine exactly what knee condition you have and therefore which exercises to perform.

Therefore it is vital to follow the exercise sequence outlined in this chapter as it is a systematic approach that will enable you to successfully self-treat your knee condition.

This chapter describes and clearly illustrates a series of exercises, and also gives you information as to **WHEN** to apply the exercises and the responses that may be expected.

It is important to remember the difference between exercising for pain relief and exercising for stiffness as you perform these exercises as described in Chapter 4.

When you are ready to begin the exercise program, **we recommend that you try each of the exercises described below first with your pain-free leg, and then cautiously attempt the same exercise with your painful leg.** In this way you can compare the pain and range of motion in both knees and use this as a baseline to monitor the progress as you perform the program to reduce the pain and restore the mobility and function in your painful knee.

If you are in significant pain or if you have injured your knee within one to two days, we recommend you refer to the section on Acute Management on page 69 in Chapter 6 before beginning this program.

It is also very important, particularly when in significant pain, to follow the postural education in Chapter 3 in an attempt to find resting positions where you are as comfortable as possible in sitting, standing and lying.

When significant pain has subsided or you have only intermittent pain, you may still feel some pain when moving your knee in certain ways. You will notice this when attempting activities that require you to straighten your leg, such as standing, walking or running; or when you are required to bend your knee, such as sitting, crouching, lifting an object from the ground or using stairs. It is likely that there is an obstruction to movement within your knee or that healing is underway within the overstretched or damaged tissues and requires motion and optimal loading to maximize this repair phase. Exercises 1 to 6 will assist with improving the range of motion and function in your knee. Exercises 7 and 8 will assist with restoring strength and endurance in the surrounding muscles and can also be used to effectively treat a condition known as anterior knee pain, where your knee has a normal range of motion yet is still painful.

The first step of the exercise program is for you to determine if there is a difference in the range of motion between your painful and pain-free knee. This will provide you with a baseline to enable you to monitor your progress as you perform the program.

To compare the range of motion between your pain-free knee and your painful knee, start by sitting upright and well back in a firm chair (Photo 28) with your feet flat on the floor.

First, try straightening the knee. This is known as knee extension. Slowly lift the foot of your **pain-free** leg and straighten your knee until you feel a firm tension at your knee and in the quadriceps muscle above your knee as it contracts (Photo 29). Straighten the knee as far as you can. Hold for a few seconds and then return your foot to the starting position. Now try the same exercise with the painful knee and compare the range of motion, and note any pain or discomfort. If you are able, you can also straighten both legs at the same time. This is another method to determine if there is a loss of extension and/or pain in your painful knee compared to your pain-free knee. Many people will find that this is the case.

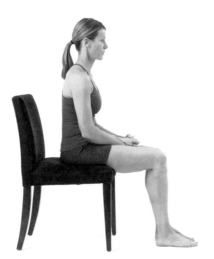

Photo 28
Sitting in chair – starting position

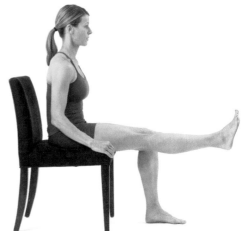

Photo 29
Active knee extension

Now, try bending your knee. This is known as knee flexion. Sit on the edge of a chair (photo 30). If you lean backward you will find it easier to perform this exercise. Slowly bend your pain-free knee up toward you, and with both hands, pull up on your leg just above your ankle. Slowly pull your heel toward your buttock until you feel a firm tension at your knee (Photo 31). If you have difficulty performing this exercise for any reason, try holding the knee with one hand and pull on the ankle with the other hand, or use a towel around your ankle if you cannot reach down that far. Bring the heel as close as possible to the buttock, hold for a few seconds, and then return your knee to the starting position.

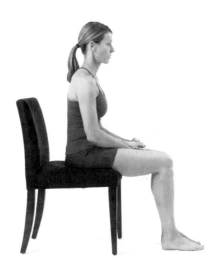

Photo 30
Sitting in chair—starting position

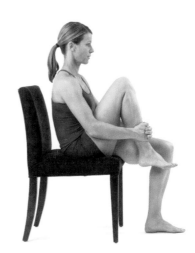

Photo 31
Knee flexion

Now cautiously try the same exercise with the painful knee and compare the range of motion, and note if there is any pain or discomfort.

If you have found that in your painful knee there is a loss of extension or flexion, or both directions, this may be the result of a previous injury, but commonly it can also occur over a period of time for no apparent reason. This reduced range of motion must be restored in order to improve your knee pain and function by carefully performing the following exercise program.

To start this process of recovery

Many people with knee pain respond to performing either knee extension exercises (Exercises 1-3) or flexion exercises (Exercises 4-6) as their first exercises.

In order to determine whether it is extension, flexion, or strengthening exercises that are going to be of benefit for you, it is very important that you observe closely any changes in your pain and range of motion during and after the exercise program. If your pain localizes to a specific area or feels better following the exercises, and it is easier to move your knee and perform your daily activities, this indicates you are performing the correct exercise. However, if your pain is no better or it is worse, your knee is less mobile following the exercise, and it is more difficult to perform your daily activities, then you are not doing the correct exercise and need to move on to the next exercise in the sequence.

It is important to be aware that as you will be repeating each exercise up to ten times, your knee may initially be uncomfortable, and it may temporarily reproduce your pain, or in some instances produce a new pain in another part of your knee. This does not mean that it is the incorrect exercise. If your knee feels improved *after* the exercise sequence, even though it was painful while performing the exercise, it was in the correct direction. *Only* if the pain steadily increases during the exercise and remains more painful *after* performing the exercise sequence on several occasions is it likely not to be the correct exercise and you need to progress on to the next exercise. In some cases it may require you to perform each exercise over 24 to 48 hours to determine if your knee pain is decreasing and movement and function is increasing.

To determine if knee extension exercises are of benefit, you need to perform Exercises 1, 2 and 3 even though there may be some temporary increase in pain, as it is necessary to ensure the possible benefits of extension have been thoroughly explored.

Again, always compare your painful leg to your pain-free leg as a useful baseline when attempting any of the following exercises.

Exercise 1: Active knee extension in sitting

This exercise helps regain the full extension in your knee and also assists in restoring the ability of your knee to perform daily activities. Exercise 1 is also a way of maintaining or increasing the strength of the ligaments, muscles and tendons around your knee.

Start by sitting upright in a firm chair (Photo 32) with your feet flat on the floor. Slowly lift the foot of your painful leg and straighten your knee until you feel a firm tension at your knee and in the quadriceps muscle as it contracts (Photo 33). Hold for a few seconds and then return your foot to the starting position. Each time you perform this movement cycle try to straighten your knee a little farther so that in the end you have reached the maximum possible knee extension. Exercise 1 should be repeated 10 times per session and the sessions should be spread evenly six to eight times throughout the day until you go to bed at night. This means you should repeat the sessions about every two hours.

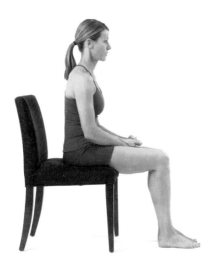

Photo 32
Sitting in chair – starting position

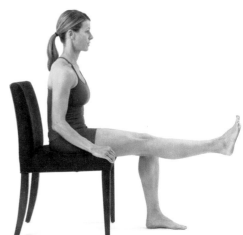

Photo 33
Active knee extension

If you find this exercise uncomfortable to perform sitting up, it can also be performed sitting on a bed or the floor with your arms supporting you and a rolled towel under your affected knee (Photo 34). Slowly lift the foot of your affected leg and straighten your knee while keeping the back of your knee on the towel until you feel a firm tension at your knee and in the quadriceps muscle as it contracts (Photo 35). Hold for a few seconds and then return your foot to the starting position. Each time you perform this movement cycle, try to brace your knee a little more so that in the end you are able to firmly brace your knee to full extension.

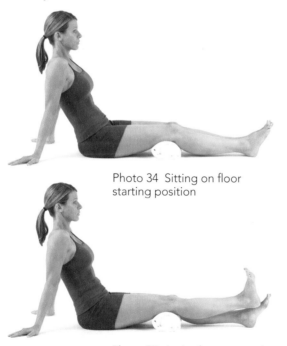

Photo 34 Sitting on floor starting position

Photo 35 Active knee extension

When you have reached the stage that either your pain reduces or you are able to straighten your knee more easily, you can progress on to Exercise 2: Knee extension in sitting, and Exercise 3: Knee extension in standing. If you perform Exercise 1 for two days without any benefit, still progress on to Exercise 2 and Exercise 3.

Exercise 2: Knee Extension in sitting

Sit in a chair and place the heel of your painful leg on a chair or stool of similar height with your knee slightly bent and foot pointing vertically (Photo 36). Now you are ready to start Exercise 2.

Let your knee relax and slowly sag so it straightens farther until you feel a firm stretch at your knee (Photo 37). Hold this position for a few seconds, and then return your knee to the starting position to release the pressure (Photo 36). Each time you perform this movement cycle, try to relax your leg and allow your knee to straighten farther so that in the end you have reached the maximum possible extension compared to your pain-free knee. Each time you repeat the exercise you must move just into the pain and then release the pressure.

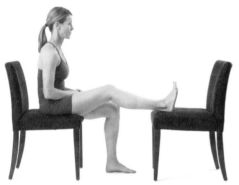

Photo 36 Extension in sitting – starting position

Exercise 2 should be repeated 10 times per session and the sessions should be spread evenly six to eight times throughout the day until you go to bed at night. This means you should repeat the sessions about every two hours.

Repeat the exercise up to ten times. Each time you repeat the exercise you must move just into the pain and then release the pressure. Once you can comfortably let your knee sag into the extension, you can progress this exercise to ensure you are getting to end range by applying an overpressure just above your knee with your hands.

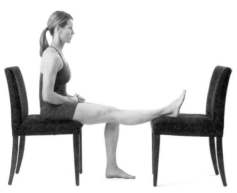

Photo 37 Extension in sitting

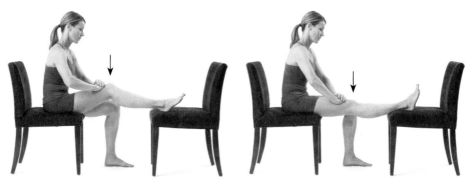

Photo 38 Extension in sitting with overpressure – starting position

Photo 39 Extension in sitting with overpressure

Starting from the same position with your foot on the chair, reach forward with both hands and place them **just above** your knee (Photo 38). Again, relax your leg and allow your knee to reach the maximum possible extension, and then slowly push your knee straight with your hands until you feel a firm stretch at your knee (Photo 39). Once you have held this position for a few seconds, release the pressure and return to the starting position (Photo 38). Repeat the exercise 10 times. Each time you perform this movement cycle try to relax your leg and allow your knee to straighten farther so that in the end you have reached the maximum possible extension. When you apply the overpressure you must move **just into the pain** and then release the pressure.

If you feel tension behind the knee, which is limiting full extension, or you have difficulty performing this exercise in this position, you can also perform the exercise with your heel on the floor or a low stool (photo 40).

Again, each time you apply the overpressure you must move **just into the pain** and then release the pressure. Continue performing the exercise for a few days. When you can comfortably perform this exercise, progress to Exercise 3: Knee extension in standing. If you perform Exercise 2 for two days without any benefit, still progress on to Exercise 3.

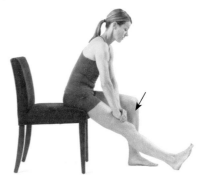

Photo 40 Extension in sitting with overpressure (foot on floor)

Exercise 3: Knee extension in standing

Stand upright and place the heel of your affected leg on a low step (Photo 41), a stool, or the floor. Let your affected knee relax and reach forward with both hands and place them just above your knee. Slowly apply a downward pressure to push your knee straight with your hands until you feel a firm stretch at your knee.

Hold for a few seconds and then return your knee to the starting position. Each time you perform this movement cycle, use your hands to push the knee straight, allowing the knee to reach the maximum possible extension. Repeat the exercise 10 times. Each time you repeat the exercise you must move just into the pain and then release the pressure.

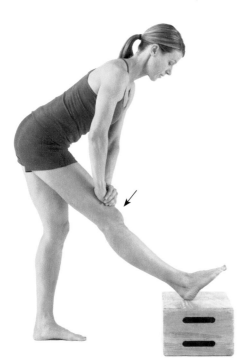

Over a few days, you will generally find that the movement begins to improve and you can progress this exercise to ensure you are getting to end range by applying a firmer overpressure. Exercise 3 should be repeated 10 times per session and the sessions should be spread evenly six to eight times throughout the day until you go to bed at night. This means you should repeat the sessions about every two hours.

Photo 41 Extension in standing with overpressure

If you are still unable to fully straighten your knee and your knee has stopped improving, it is necessary to progress Exercise 3 further by performing this exercise with your knee turned outward, known as external rotation (photo 42), or inward, known as internal rotation (photo 43). One of these variations may be required to enable Exercise 3 to be more effective. If that is the case, then this variation of knee extension is the one that should be used. If your pain is on the inside of your knee, try rotating the foot outward initially. If this does not increase your knee extension over a few repetitions, try it with your foot turned inward. If the pain is on the outside of your knee, perform this exercise sequence starting with your foot turned inward.

Again, this variation of Exercise 3 should be repeated 10 times per session and the sessions should be spread evenly six to eight times throughout the day until you go to bed at night. This means you should repeat the sessions about every two hours.

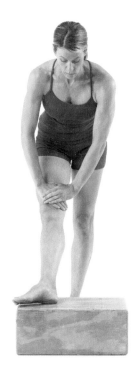

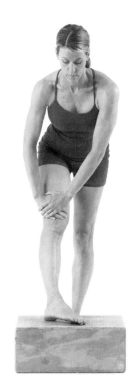

Photo 42
External rotation

Photo 43
Internal rotation

Review your progress

If you have found your knee pain has improved and your movement and function has increased after performing Exercises 1, 2 and 3, continue to perform Exercise 3 for up to a further one or two weeks until your knee is pain-free or your progress has plateaued. Once your knee is pain-free, perform Exercise 4, 5 and 6 to restore the normal range of flexion to your affected knee.

However, if you have performed Exercises 1, 2 and 3 over several days without noticing any improvement in your knee pain or your ability to bend or straighten your knee, it is necessary to perform Exercises 4, 5 and 6 to determine if knee flexion exercises will reduce your pain and increase your movement and function.

Exercise 4: Knee flexion in sitting

Start by sitting upright in a firm chair (Photo 44). If you sit forward on the edge of the chair and lean backward, you will find it easier to perform this exercise. Slowly bend your knee up toward you, and with both hands pull up on your leg just above your ankle. Slowly pull your heel toward your buttock until you feel a firm tension at your knee (Photo 45). If you have difficulty performing this exercise for any reason, try holding the knee with one hand and pull on the ankle with the other hand, or use a towel around your ankle if you cannot reach down that far. Bring the heel as close as possible to the buttock, hold for a few seconds, and then return your knee to the starting position (Photo 44).

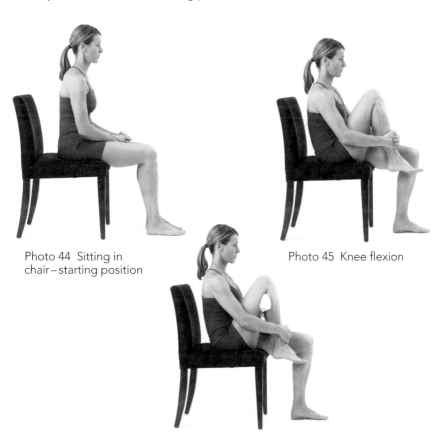

Photo 44 Sitting in chair–starting position

Photo 45 Knee flexion

Photo 46 Knee flexion with towel behind knee

Repeat the exercise 10 times. If there is no pain or loss of movement compared to your pain-free knee, you can progress to exercise 5. But if there is discomfort, each time you repeat the exercise you must move just into the pain and then release the pressure. Over a few days you will generally find that the movement begins to improve and you can progress this exercise to ensure you are getting to maximum flexion by applying a firmer overpressure. Hold for a few seconds and then return your knee to the starting position. Each time you perform this movement cycle, try to bend your knee a little farther so that in the end you have reached the maximum possible flexion over 10 repetitions.

If you find your knee is too uncomfortable when initially attempting to perform this exercise, place a small rolled towel behind your knee (Photo 46) to relieve the discomfort and perform the exercise again. Push the towel into the back of the knee with your fingers while flexing to keep it in place. Once this exercise is comfortable to perform, remove the towel to ensure you are getting the maximum possible flexion. Exercise 4 should be repeated 10 times per session and the sessions should be spread evenly six to eight times throughout the day until you go to bed at night. This means you should repeat the sessions about every two hours.

Once you are able to perform Exercise 4 comfortably, progress to Exercise 5.

Exercise 5: Knee flexion in standing

Stand upright and place the foot of your affected leg on a chair or stool (Photo 47). If you feel unsteady, place a hand on the chair for balance. Let your affected knee relax and slowly lean forward, pushing your buttock toward your heel until you feel a firm stretch at your knee (Photo 48).

Hold for a few seconds and then return your knee to the starting position (Photo 47). Repeat the exercise up to 10 times. Each time you repeat the exercise, you must move just into the pain and then release the pressure. Each time you perform this movement cycle, try to bend your knee a little further so that in the end you have reached the maximum possible flexion over approximately 10 repetitions.

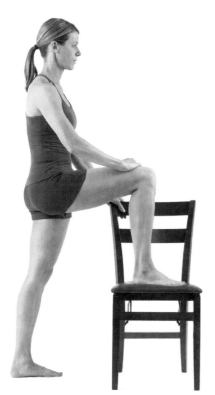

Photo 47 Standing foot on chair
–starting position

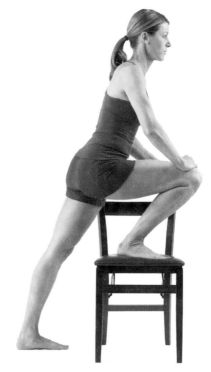

Photo 48 Knee flexion

Exercise 5 should be repeated 10 times per session and the sessions should be spread evenly six to eight times throughout the day until you go to bed at night. This means you should repeat the sessions about every two hours.

Your pain should decrease over a period of several days, or up to a few weeks, as this movement improves. You should be able to bend your affected leg back as comfortably as your pain-free leg. If you find your knee is too uncomfortable when attempting to perform this exercise, place a small rolled towel behind your knee (Photo 49) to relieve the discomfort and perform the exercise again. Push the towel into the back of the knee with your fingers while flexing to keep it in place. Once this exercise is comfortable to perform, remove the towel to ensure you are getting the maximum possible flexion.

Once you are able to perform Exercise 5 comfortably, progress to Exercise 6.

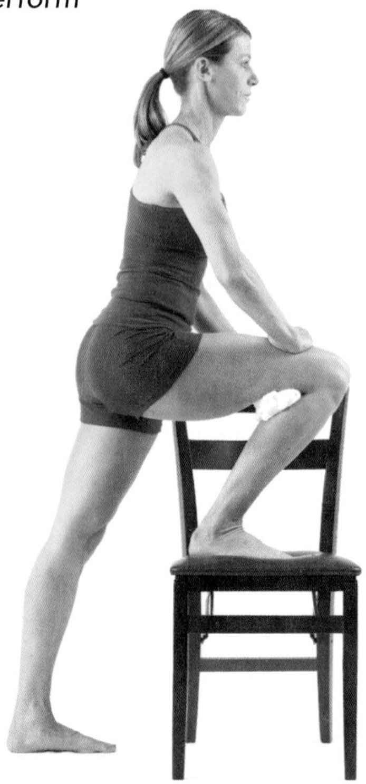

Photo 49 Knee flexion with towel

Exercise 6: Knee flexion in kneeling

Start cautiously with this exercise, but do not be frightened to attempt it, as it can be a very effective progression from the previous flexion exercises to ensure you recover full flexion in your knee. However, if you find kneeling too uncomfortable to tolerate, or your knee feels worse following this exercise, stop this exercise and go back to performing the flexion in either sitting or standing (Exercises 4 and 5), and in most cases you will achieve the same outcome.

Start on your hands and knees with a cushion or pillow under your knees for comfort (Photo 50). Let your affected knee relax and slowly sit back toward your heels until you feel a firm stretch at your knee (Photo 51). Keep your hands on the floor in front of you, taking some of the weight at first until you get confident with this exercise. Once you have held this position for a few seconds, release the pressure and return to the starting position (Photo 50). Each time you perform this movement cycle, try to bend your knee a little farther so that in the end you have reached the maximum possible flexion over 6 to 10 repetitions. Once you can comfortably kneel back on your heels (Photo 51), you can progress to lifting your hands off the floor and sitting on your heels for a few seconds (Photo 52) before returning to the starting position (Photo 50). Repeat the exercise up to 10 times. Each time you repeat the exercise, you must move just into the pain and then release the pressure.

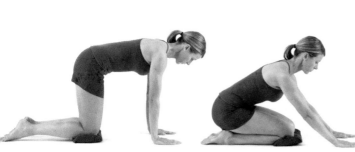

Photo 50 Kneeling on all fours – starting position

Photo 51 Kneeling back on heels

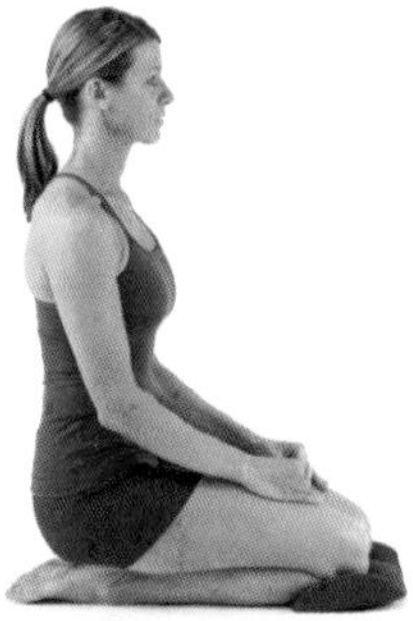

Photo 52 Sitting back fully on heels

Exercise 6 should be repeated 6 to 10 times per session and the sessions should be spread evenly four to six times throughout the day until you go to bed at night. This means you should repeat the sessions about every three hours.

Your pain should decrease over a period of several days, or up to a few weeks, as this movement improves. You should be able to bend your affected leg back as comfortably as your pain-free leg.

Review your progress

If you found your knee has responded to flexion exercises (Exercises 4, 5 and 6), continue to perform Exercise 5 or Exercise 6 for up to a further one to two weeks until your knee is pain-free or your progress has plateaued. If flexion exercises were the ones that reduced your pain and extension exercises were not helpful initially, it is still necessary to try working the extension exercises back into the program. You should have healed enough to do them now. Start gradually and always do a set of one of the flexion exercises after extension. *The rule is to always finish with the exercise that corrected the initial painful problem.*

Painful problems are often rapidly improved as you remove the obstruction inside the knee. However, stiffness rather than pain is more due to tight scar tissue, which must gradually be lengthened over a longer period of time.

Therefore, if you feel only stiffness rather than pain on performing Exercise 3 or Exercise 5 or 6, you should continue to perform these exercises, but apply more overpressure at the end of each movement. By exercising in this way you achieve movement to the maximum possible degree. In most cases, you will restore normal function within six weeks.

Once you have restored the normal range of motion to your affected knee and are able to perform Exercises 1 to 6 fully with no pain compared to your pain-free knee, you will usually find that you no longer have knee pain and have regained the functional use of your affected knee.

However, do not forget the important postural education in Chapter 3 to prevent the onset of your pain at rest.

If you are completely symptom-free, follow the *When you have no pain or stiffness guidelines on page 66* to prevent recurrence of knee problems.

No response or benefit

If, after performing Exercises 1 to 6 for a few weeks, you still experience knee pain on activities that require you to bend your knee, such as prolonged sitting, walking up or down stairs or hills, or kneeling or crouching, it is necessary to progress on to strengthening the ligaments, muscles and tendons around your knee. If this is the case, you should commence with Exercise 7 below.

As described earlier in Chapter 3, on page 34, **anterior knee pain** is one of the conditions that can be challenging to treat successfully and requires a program of carefully performed weight-bearing exercises to result in a successful outcome. If you have been diagnosed with anterior knee pain, we recommend you first perform Exercises 1 to 6 thoroughly as described in this chapter to ensure your knee is moving completely freely and that a loss of movement is not the underlying cause of the pain.

Exercises 7 and 8 are designed to increase the weight-bearing capacity, strength, elasticity and function of the injured tendons around your knee in order to perform daily activities more easily. Start cautiously with a few repetitions through a small range of motion, and gradually increase the number of repetitions. You may feel some discomfort in the muscles around your knee initially, which can be expected, but this should not worsen as you repeat this exercise. Any pain produced from performing these exercises should go away within 15 minutes of completing the exercise session, otherwise you are exercising too vigorously.

Exercise 7: Knee strengthening in standing, two-legged knee bend

Stand upright with your feet placed shoulder width apart, a chair or stool behind you, and an open door in front of you where you are able to grasp both door handles for support (Photo 53). Keep your feet flat on the floor, and slowly sit back toward the chair until you feel a firm tension in the muscles around your knee (Photo 54). Start with a small range of motion and do not sit on the chair. Hold this position for a few seconds, and then return to the starting position.

Each time you perform this movement cycle, try to keep your knees pointing forward, and lower your hips farther — until your buttocks are almost touching the back of the chair — so that in the end you are able to perform this amount of controlled knee flexion with no knee pain. Exercise 7 should be repeated 10 to 15 times per session two times a day — once in the morning and again in the afternoon or evening. **Each time you repeat the exercise you must move just into the pain and then release the pressure by returning to the starting position.**

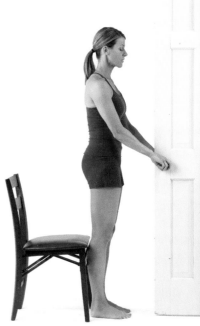

Photo 53
Squatting holding door – starting position

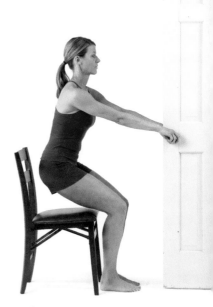

Photo 54
Squatting holding door

Once you can perform this exercise without difficulty over a few days or weeks, progress the exercise by performing the knee bends without holding on to the door handle (Photos 55 and 56).

As your ability to perform this exercise improves, you can steadily progress the number of repetitions until you are performing up to three sets of 15 repetitions twice a day. By exercising this way, you place the appropriate loading required to stimulate a recovery in the affected structures around your knee. Your pain should decrease over a few weeks as your knee regains its ability to withstand weight-bearing activities.

If you can perform Exercise 7 without difficulty, or after two or three weeks your knee pain is not decreasing when performing bent knee activities like rising from a chair or going downstairs, progress on to Exercise 8.

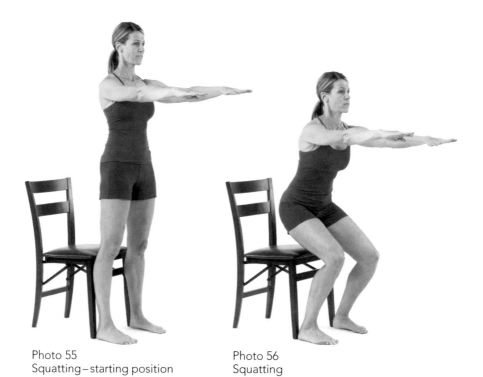

Photo 55
Squatting – starting position

Photo 56
Squatting

Exercise 8: Knee strengthening in standing, one-legged knee bend

A more advanced functional strengthening exercise is to progress to a single-leg knee bend. **This exercise is particularly important if you have anterior knee pain.**

Stand upright on your affected leg along the edge of a step, or use a box, with a chair or rail beside you for support (Photo 57). *Slowly* bend your affected knee so the foot of your pain-free leg is lowered below the level of the step until you feel a firm tension in the muscles around your knee (Photo 58). As you perform this exercise, keep the center of your knee pointing forward (Photos 59 and 60). Hold this position for a few seconds, and then return to the starting position. The lowering phase is the most important and should take 3-5 seconds each repetition.

Each time you perform this movement cycle, start with a *small arc of motion, keep your balance* and try to lower your foot closer to the ground, but *do not touch the ground,* so that in the end you are able to perform this amount of controlled knee flexion with no knee pain.

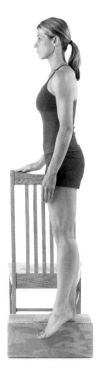

Photo 57
Standing on box –
starting position

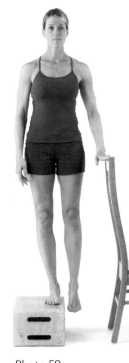

Photo 59
Standing on box –
starting position

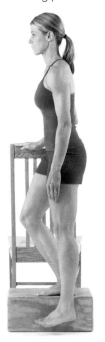

Photo 58
Bending knee

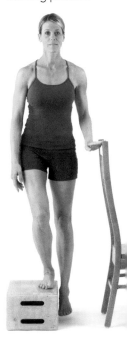

Photo 60
Bending knee

Exercise 8 should be repeated 10 to 15 times per session two times a day—once in the morning and again in the afternoon or evening. Each time you repeat the exercise you must move just into the pain and then release the pressure by returning to the starting position.

Again, your pain should decrease over a few weeks as your knee regains its function performing activities that require your knee to take your body weight while bending.

This exercise can be further progressed by performing the exercise without holding onto the chair (Photo 61 and 62), and also by bending the knee farther.

Keep the center of your knee pointing forward, and *slowly* bend your affected knee so the foot of your pain-free leg is lowered below the level of the step until you feel a firm tension in the muscles around your knee. Hold this position for a few seconds, and then return to the starting position. Each time you perform this movement cycle, start with a *small arc of motion, keep your balance* and try to lower your foot closer to the ground, *but do not touch the ground,* so that in the end you are able to perform this amount of controlled knee flexion with no knee pain over approximately 10 to 15 repetitions. Progress to

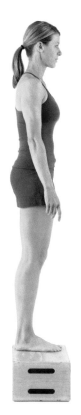

Photo 61
Standing on box

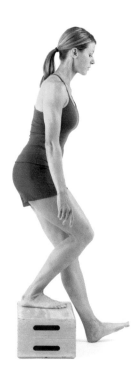

Photo 62
Stepping down off box

allowing your heel (not toes) to lightly touch the ground as you go down. Placing a book under the heel of your painful leg, so that your heel is higher than your toes, also increases the amount of load on the knee as a further progression.

As your ability to perform this exercise improves, you can steadily progress the number of repetitions until you are performing up to three sets of 15 repetitions twice a day. By exercising this way, you place the optimal loading required to stimulate a recovery in the affected structures around your knee.

In the case of anterior knee pain, we recommend you perform Exercises 7 and 8 for up to six weeks to determine if the exercises are of benefit in reducing or abolishing your pain. A gradual decrease in pain when you perform activities such as going down hills, stairs, crouching or jumping indicates your knee pain is improving. In most cases, the result eventually is a good recovery, however, progress can be slow, and some cases gradually improve over several months. Try to get to the point where your affected knee is as strong as your pain-free, or less painful leg, and be prepared to resume the exercise program if you feel your pain returning.

To prevent the recurrence of anterior knee pain, it is crucial to maintain your ability to perform Exercise 7 and Exercise 8. Also, it is necessary to continue to adopt good postures and positional habits for the knee as described in Chapter 3.

If you continue to have knee pain and a loss of function that is not resolving, we recommend that you contact a healthcare professional who is fully qualified to provide the McKenzie Method®. These are members of the McKenzie Institute International who hold the Credentialing Certificate or the Diploma in Mechanical Diagnosis & Therapy®. A clinician in your area can be located via the McKenzie Institute International website www.mckenziemdt.org.

When you have no pain or stiffness

Many people with knee problems have lengthy spells in which they experience little or no pain. If you have ever had one or more episodes of knee pain, you should start the exercise program even though you may be pain-free at the moment. However, in this situation it is not necessary to do all the exercises or to exercise every two hours.

To prevent recurrence of knee problems, you should perform Exercise 3: Knee extension in standing (Photo 63) followed by Exercise 5: Knee flexion in standing (Photo 64) two times a day to ensure you maintain your knee's range of motion. These exercises could also be performed sitting, if this is more suitable for you (Exercises 2 and 4).

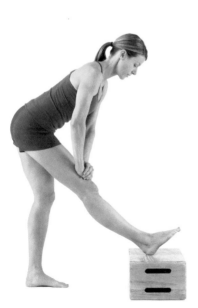

Photo 63 Knee extension in standing

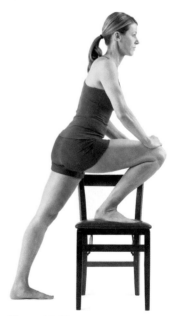

Photo 64 Knee flexion in standing

If either Exercise 7: Knee strengthening, two-legged knee bend (Photo 65) or Exercise 8: Knee strengthening, one-legged knee bend (Photo 66) has been the exercise sequence that has relieved your knee symptoms, perform these exercises instead.

Furthermore, whenever you feel pain developing during activity or work, or while sitting, you should perform these exercises. It is important that you watch your knee postures at all times and never again let postural stresses be the cause of knee pain. These exercises will have very little or no effect if you constantly fall back into your previous poor knee postures and prolonged bent knee positions. While it may be advisable to exercise in the manner described on the previous pages for the rest of your life, it is absolutely essential that you develop and maintain good postural habits.

As it takes only a few minutes to perform one session of these exercises, lack of time should never be used as an excuse for not being able to do these exercises.

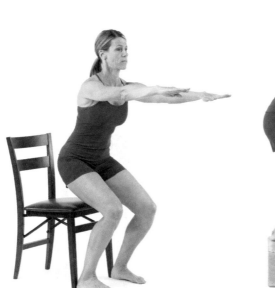
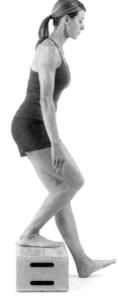

Photo 65 Squatting   Photo 66 Stepping down

Yoga, Pilates, Tai Chi and martial arts are activities that specifically promote postural awareness while also using exercises that will ensure the knees and legs are put through a wide range of motion.

A graduated increase in activities that generally improve your fitness should also be considered. Even a regular walking, cycling or stationary bicycle program will assist in maintaining leg mobility, whereas appropriately structured gym programs and aerobics or fitness classes are examples of activities that will specifically assist with flexibility and strength at and around the knee. Further specific strategies to prevent recurrence are covered in more detail in Chapter 6.

Recurrence

At the first sign of recurrence of knee pain, you should immediately perform the exercises that have previously helped you.

If your pain is already too severe to tolerate these exercises or if they fail to reduce the pain, you must review the advice provided under the acute management section of Chapter 6. This will help you to determine when you can return to Exercise 1: Active knee extension, and then gradually work through the exercise sequence again. Again, you must pay extra attention to your knee posture, regularly perform postural correction, and maintain the correct posture as much as you can when sitting, standing and lying.

Chapter 6: Acute Management and Prevention of Recurrence

Acute management

If you have injured your knee within the past few days by twisting it or receiving a blow, it is possible you have injured a ligament, meniscus or joint surface and triggered an inflammatory response, which is the body's response to injury. This inflammatory response can also be triggered by suddenly overstressing or overloading the knee without a specific injury or incident.

The knee will be painful at rest and on moving it or attempting to take weight on that leg. It may appear warm, and often there will be some swelling.

In the early stage, it is necessary to reduce the effects of the injury by limiting any bleeding, swelling and pain through applying the regime of Protect, Optimal Loading, Ice, Compression and Elevation (POLICE).

Protecting your knee from further damage by avoiding any activity that increases your pain and swelling is important for the first 24-48 hours. If you are limping when walking, the use of a walking stick will help when you have to walk short distances (Photo 67) in order to walk more evenly and provide the optimal loading rather than full weight bearing.

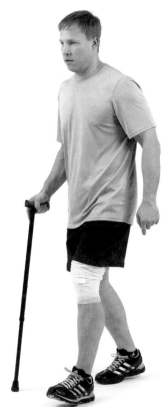

Photo 67 Using a walking stick for short distances

Elevation of the knee above the level of your heart when possible will limit the development of further swelling at your injury site (Photo 68). Apply a cold pack to your knee over the painful region for up to 15 minutes every three hours. To prevent an ice burn, place a damp towel or a thin layer of cooking or baby oil between your skin and the ice pack (Photo 69).

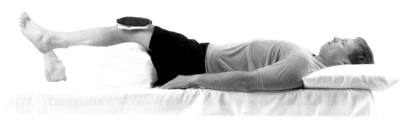

Photo 68 Applying an ice pack in elevation

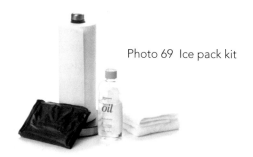

Photo 69 Ice pack kit

To limit the swelling at your knee, apply an elastic bandage between ice pack sessions and wear day and night (Photo 70), elevating the leg whenever possible.

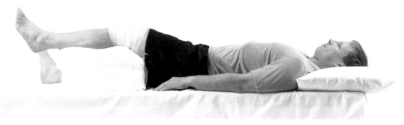

Photo 70 Elevating the leg while bandaged

After 24 hours of applying POLICE treatment, we recommend you cautiously commence the exercise program in Chapter 5 and follow the advice carefully. This will allow you to judge the optimal loading and also the correct direction of movement for your knee. Continue with the application of ice and compression for up to one week, as required, until the pain and swelling has reduced.

If it is too painful to perform the exercise program, continue with POLICE for a further 24 hours then try again. If your knee is too painful to commence the exercise program after 48 hours, we recommend you consult your doctor or physical therapist.

Prevention of recurrence

In earlier chapters we have discussed a specific exercise regime to follow to decrease pain, and increase flexibility and strength in your knee. However, we also discussed that exercises alone are only a part of the solution, and in order to prevent or minimize further episodes, it is very important to address the other aggravating factors that contribute to your knee pain.

The most important thing for most people is to be more active — with walking, swimming or running, for example — and often lose some body weight. Cycling is another good option for many people, but bear in mind that you are still in a sitting position, and if you already sit for long periods in other areas of your life, other recreational activities will get other parts of your body moving more.

This chapter aims to give you simple strategies to assist with changes of lifestyle that are an important part of breaking the cycle of recurrent knee pain, and covers these main areas:

1. Interrupt prolonged sitting and standing postures regularly.

2. Increase your walking.

3. Increase your general fitness.

4. Improve your balance.

5. Lose weight.

Most of these strategies are designed to be used in conjunction with the exercise program described in this book to reduce the pain and improve the endurance, strength and function of your knee. Any movement or exercise is generally beneficial provided you choose activities that don't make your knee pain worse, but as a general rule — start cautiously. Some knee discomfort while exercising may be expected as long as it goes away afterward. If you do over-exercise your knee and create more pain or swelling, refer back to the acute management section at the beginning of this chapter.

1. Interrupt prolonged sitting and standing postures regularly

As we have discussed in Chapter 3, many of us have a sedentary job or lifestyle, and the hours pass before we realize that we have not changed position, or we develop discomfort or pain that reminds us to move. This can also occur less frequently with prolonged standing. The key is to move regularly before pain develops by building movement into your daily routines. There are several ways you can achieve this:

At work:

- Use a printer that you have to walk to, rather than one directly by your desk.

- Walk the long way to the café or lunch room during your work breaks.

- Set your software or cell phone to sound an alarm every 20 minutes or so to remind you to get up and stretch your legs with a short walk.

- If it's difficult to get up, as in a plane or car, try to stretch your legs out while sitting.

At home:

- Leave the remote control at the opposite side of the room to your favorite seat so that you have to get up and move when you want to use the remote control.

- If you are watching TV, get up and move about every time the advertisements come on.

- Avoid a low chair. Ensure you sit in a firm chair at a height from which you can stand without too much effort—using your legs as much as possible, with minimal assistance from your arms, if required.

- Do a few leg stretches in bed when you wake up or before going to sleep.

- When on the phone, stand up rather than sit, or if possible walk around.

2. Increase your walking

Increasing your general level of walking is probably the single most important way of increasing your strength, endurance and balance in order to prevent or minimize recurrent knee pain. First increase the number of minutes spent walking. These can be in one session, or accumulated over the day. Later, you should increase the speed and even add some hills, being particularly cautious about adding in too much walking or hiking downhill initially.

A good goal is 20-30 minutes of brisk walking, 4-5 days per week. If your knee is painful or you are unfit, you may well need to start with less and let your body gradually adapt over several weeks. Do not increase your walking by more than 10% from one session to the next. For example, if you are able to walk for 20 minutes, progress to 22 minutes. Larger increases overstress the body and can aggravate your knee pain. What you do not want is to cause more pain that will put you off further exercise — otherwise, you will return to the same cycle of losing fitness, putting on weight and continuing to have knee pain.

Ways to increase walking:

- Park your car at the far end of the parking lot rather than taking the closest parking space to your destination. This is particularly true on a long car journey when you have pulled in for a break or coffee, etc.

- Get off the bus one stop earlier than usual and walk the rest of the way to your destination.

- Use the steps or stairs rather than the elevator or escalator — for example, at the shopping mall.

- Use your meal break at work for a walk, or walk the long way to your favorite or usual eating place.

- Begin a regular walking program, preferably with someone such as a family member or friend to keep you motivated. Or join a local walking group.

- Buy or adopt a dog that you will have to take out for walks every day.

- Wear shoes that are comfortable and supportive. Try to walk on grass or asphalt rather than concrete, but be careful with uneven surfaces, which can be tough on the joints.

- Take a light at night to see and be seen.

- While walking, use the time for listening to music or podcasts, learning a language or listening to an audio book.

- Walking in a swimming pool is another good way to get started on a walking routine if your knees are painful initially. Walking in waist deep water reduces load through the knee by 50%.

3. Increase your fitness

Once you are comfortable with a walking program, you may feel confident to gradually increase your general fitness by adding in other pursuits—either by gradually returning to previous recreational activities or taking up new interests. But start cautiously with whatever you choose, and gradually increase the intensity and the frequency. If you are over 55 years of age, or have underlying health conditions, we recommend that you consult with your own doctor or healthcare professional about your exercise plans.

Ways to increase fitness:

- Start a graduated swimming, running or fitness routine, or join a local group or fitness club in your area.

- Get a bicycle, mountain bike or stationary bicycle, and start a cycling routine. Or join a cycling club in your area.

- Resume activities that you have enjoyed in the past, such as fitness classes, dancing or golf, for example.

- Take up ANY ACTIVITY that you enjoy doing, have enjoyed in the past, or have always thought about doing.

- Join a local gym and get a supervised graduated fitness program. Be cautious with any deep squatting or squats with weights if you are not used to it.

Injury Prevention Tips:

- We recommend you be able to walk comfortably for one hour before you consider higher impact activities, such as jogging, tennis, or football that involve some running.

- Running is more risky for injury if you are overweight, and you will need to start more cautiously, following these injury prevention tips even more carefully.

- Initially, avoid running down hills as significant increased loading is placed on your knees.

- Take time to warm up and cool down: The best way to warm up for an activity is to do that activity gently for the first five minutes. A cool down at the end, again doing the activity gently as you gradually slow down, keeps blood pumping back to the heart and vital organs as you recover.

- Give your body a chance to recover from exercise by taking days off. If you do high impact activities, be cautious with activity on the following day. Either rest or just do some easy walking or cycling to assist with the recovery.

- Varying your activities has been shown to reduce overuse problems. Walk some days, and swim or cycle other days. If weather or environmental factors are a problem, consider using a treadmill, elliptical or cross trainer machine, or a stationary bicycle.

- Proper footwear is also important for most people, especially if walking or running on hard surfaces. And, if possible, run on grass in a park or a trail in the woods rather than concrete, as the loading stress through the knees is significantly less.

4. Improve your balance

There are simple ways to specifically stimulate the balance reactions in your knee joint — either when standing still or when on the move. Exercises 7 and 8 are effective in improving your balance as well as your strength, and we give some other suggestions below. Further specific ways of improving your balance are Tai Chi classes or falls prevention programs run by community groups or health professionals.

Simple exercises:

- Balance on one leg — when brushing your teeth, talking on the phone, or standing doing a task at a table or counter (e.g., a cooking task or washing the dishes) (Photo 71).

- Progress this by closing your eyes, rising onto your toes, or going into a slight squat on that leg.

- Sometimes go up or down stairs very slowly to challenge your strength and balance.

- Try walking one foot in front of the other like a tightrope walker down your hallway, with arms outstretched to touch the walls if your balance is unsteady (Photo 72).

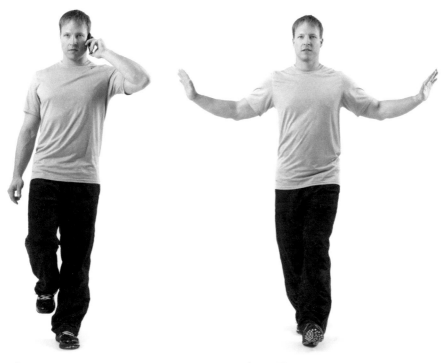

Photo 71
Balance on one leg

Photo 72
Walking like a tightrope walker

Before starting to use poles for walking and hiking consider whether you really need to use such walking aids. They are promoted as helping you feel more stable on uneven ground, or decreasing the load on the knee, particularly when walking downhill. But actually the opposite is required.

It is better to improve your balance and knee function by gradually increasing the load on your knee with exercise, rather than over-protecting the knee and decreasing the load as a long-term solution. Once you start using a stick or pole, you will become increasingly reliant on it.

5. Weight loss

Losing weight is achievable for most people. But, maintaining that weight loss is more difficult. Do NOT diet. Dieting is a short-term strategy, usually doomed to fail in the long-term. Strive for a healthier lifestyle with moderate changes you can live with long-term. To lose a significant amount of weight healthily takes 6-24 months. People who lose weight quickly tend to regain it with adverse effects on the metabolism. Aiming to lose a pound (half a kilo) a week on a consistent basis is a reasonable and obtainable goal. Portion control has been shown to be more effective when combined with exercise.

As mentioned in Chapter 3, we recommend you seek advice from your doctor or physician, or attend a recognized weight loss program should you have underlying health issues or seek to lose a significant amount of weight.

Top tips to lose weight:

- Eat less each meal (smaller portions) — even if you do not immediately change the food you are eating. Reduce the size of your meals by 25% or stop eating when you are 75% full. Within 20 minutes, the food will expand in your body and you will feel satisfied.

- Researchers have found overweight people eat more quickly. Slow down and give the food a chance to register and expand in your stomach.

- Stop unhealthy snacks (e.g., chocolate, sweet snacks, chips).

- Eat a more balanced diet including healthy, low-fat options and a greater percent of fruit and vegetables.

- Drink more water, but less alcohol, soda pops, and fizzy drinks, which have a high sugar content.

- Order less food in restaurants. Split a meal with a friend, order fewer courses, or ask for a container for you to take away any excess food when you are full.

- Do not shop when hungry. You will make poor choices. Avoid having unhealthy food in the house.

Conclusion

The key thing to consider is that changes to your lifestyle and general fitness need to be gradually implemented in order to be sustainable. However, by following the instructions and information in this book you have every opportunity to participate in an active healthy lifestyle in order to remain pain-free, or minimize further episodes of knee pain. Should you require, or would prefer, to have a McKenzie assessment before commencing any of the exercises described in Chapter 5, or the fitness strategies discussed in this chapter, we recommend that you contact a healthcare professional who is fully qualified to provide the McKenzie Method®. These are members of the McKenzie Institute International who hold the Credentialing Certificate or the Diploma in Mechanical Diagnosis & Therapy®. A clinician in your area can be located via the McKenzie Institute International website www.mckenziemdt.org.

References

Bennell K, Hinman R (2011) A review of the clinical evidence for exercise in osteoarthritis of the hip and knee. **Journal of Science and Medicine in Sport** 14, 4–9

Bolgla L, Boling (2011) An Update for the Conservative Management of Patellofemoral Pain Syndrome: A Systematic Review of the Literature from 2000 to 2010. **International Journal of Sports Physical Therapy** 6, 2, 112-125.

Chakravarty E, Hubert H, Lingala V, Zatarain E (2008) Long Distance Running and Knee Osteoarthritis: A Prospective Study. **American Journal of Preventative Medicine** 35, 2, 133–138

Goulston LM, Kiran A, Javaid MK, Soni A, White KM, Hart DJ, Spector TD, Arden NK. (2011) Obesity predicts knee pain over 14 years in women, independent of radiographic changes. **Arthritis Care Research** (Hoboken).

Logerstedt D, Snyder-Mackler L, Ritter R, Axe M (2010) Knee Pain and Mobility Impairments: Meniscal and Articular Cartilage Lesions Clinical Practice Guidelines Linked to the International Classification of Functioning, Disability, and Health from the Orthopaedic Section of the American Physical Therapy Association **Journal of Orthopedic Sports Physical Therapy** 40, 6, A1-A35.

The McKenzie Institute International

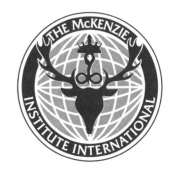

The McKenzie Institute International
Head Office website
www.mckenziemdt.org

Includes information about:
- Robin McKenzie
- The McKenzie Method of Mechanical Diagnosis and Therapy
- The McKenzie Institute International
- The McKenzie Institute's Education Program

Can help you find:
- Certified McKenzie Clinics
- Diplomaed and Credentialed McKenzie therapists
- Your local branch

The McKenzie Institute International Head Office
3 Alexander Road, PO Box 2026,
Raumati Beach 5255, New Zealand
Website: www.mckenziemdt.org
Email: mckinst@xtra.co.nz
Phone: **+64 4 299-6645** Fax: **+64 4 299-7010**

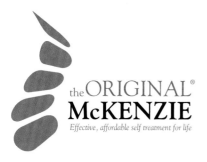

the ORIGINAL®
McKENZIE
Effective, affordable self treatment for life

The Original McKenzie® Products

Available online at OPTP.com or by calling 1-800-367-7393

Treat Your Own Back™

This worldwide best-selling book is designed to reduce and eliminate lower back pain and sciatica. It offers do-it-yourself relief through postural changes, ergonomics and simple exercises.
ITEM #802-9

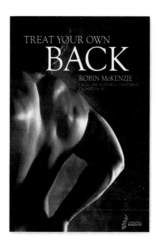

Treat Your Own Back™ DVD

Based on the best-selling book for the self-treatment of back pain and sciatica, this DVD illustrates the McKenzie Method® exercise program of extension, flexion and acute pain techniques.
ITEM #9009DVD

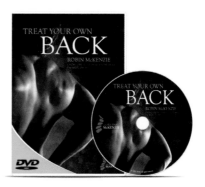

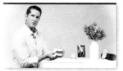
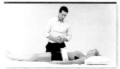

Why McKenzie Method® Works For Your Back DVD

This DVD presents the story of one man's back pain treatment journey. It is designed to provide an overview of the causes of lower back pain and how the McKenzie Method® treats it.
ITEM #9011DVD

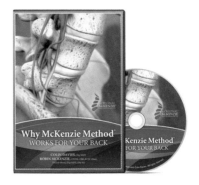

Treat Your Own Neck™

For those with persistent neck pain, this book offers a step-by-step guide to self-treatment through awareness, education and easy-to-perform McKenzie Method® exercises.
ITEM #803-5

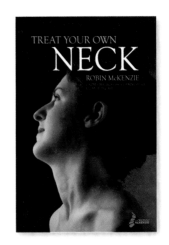

Treat Your Own Shoulder™

This book teaches the importance of stretching and demonstrates how regular practice of proper positioning helps treat and prevent shoulder area pain. Self-treatment techniques and exercises are illustrated and can easily be performed in the home.
ITEM #805

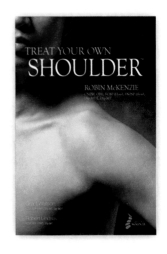

Treat Your Own Back™ and Treat Your Own Neck™ Spanish Edition

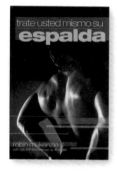
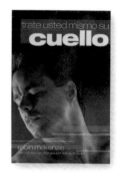

The best-selling back and neck education and self-treatment books as described previously, translated in Spanish for Spanish language readers.

ITEM #804SP (Treat Your Own Back™) ITEM #803-2SP (Treat Your Own Neck™)

The Original McKenzie® Lumbar Roll™

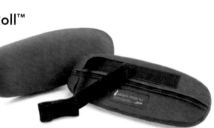

Ideal lumbar roll companion in the car, at the office or for use with any seat that does not provide adequate lumbar support. The built-in strap secures the lumbar roll to most chair backs or it can be used around the waist.

Standard Density ITEM #701 or Firm Density ITEM #702

The Original McKenzie® SuperRoll™

A low-profile lumbar support with a beveled design featuring high-resiliency and pre-compressed foam. The adjustable, removable strap easily adheres to the seat of your car or truck.

ITEM #708

The Original McKenzie® Early Compliance™ Lumbar Roll™

Smaller lumbar roll that is perfect
for youth, petite persons or
those with acute discomfort
that cannot tolerate a larger
lumbar roll. Can be attached to most
chair backs or used around the waist.
ITEM #704

The Original McKenzie® SlimLine™ Lumbar Support

A slimmer back cushion option
measuring only 2½" deep with
the shape of a crescent moon.
The SlimLine is ideal for elderly
or petite people and those who
cannot tolerate larger, more intrusive supports.
ITEM #705

Licensed Distributor

United States and Canada:

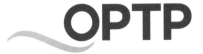

TOOLS FOR FITNESS. KNOWLEDGE FOR HEALTH.

3800 Annapolis Lane N, Suite 165
P.O. Box 47009
Minneapolis, MN 55447-0009 USA
1-800-367-7393
www.optp.com